THE BIG BOOK OF
FAMILY EYE CARE

THE BIG BOOK OF FAMILY EYE CARE

JOE DI GIROLAMO

WWW.EYECAREBOOK.COM

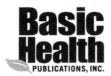

Basic Health
PUBLICATIONS, INC.

The information contained in this book is based upon the research and personal and professional experiences of the authors. It is not intended as a substitute for consulting with your physician or other healthcare provider. Any attempt to diagnose and treat an illness should be done under the direction of a healthcare professional.

The publisher does not advocate the use of any particular healthcare protocol but believes the information in this book should be available to the public. The publisher and authors are not responsible for any adverse effects or consequences resulting from the use of the suggestions, preparations, or procedures discussed in this book. Should the reader have any questions concerning the appropriateness of any procedures or preparation mentioned, the authors and the publisher strongly suggest consulting a professional healthcare advisor.

Basic Health Publications, Inc.
28812 Top of the World Drive
Laguna Beach, CA 92651
949-715-7327 • www.basichealthpub.com

Library of Congress Cataloging-in-Publication Data
Di Girolamo, Joe (Joseph)
 The big book of family eye care : a contemporary reference for vision and eye health / Joe Di Girolamo.
  p. cm.
 Includes bibliographical references and index.
 ISBN 978-1-59120-277-6
 1. Eye—Care and hygiene. 2. Ophthalmology—Popular works.
3. Optometry—Popular works. I. Title.

 RE51.D5   2010
 617.7—dc22
                                                2010044649

Watermarked eye images copyright © Eyemaginations, Inc. Reproduced by permission.

Editor: John Anderson
Typesetting/Book design: Gary A. Rosenberg
Cover design: Kristen Perkins

Printed in the United States of America

10   9   8   7   6   5   4   3   2   1

Contents

I dedicate this book to my dad,
Michael Di Girolamo, O.D., F.A.A.O.,
the perpetual encourager.

The ancient proverb says that "the eyes are the
window to the soul." Though we are doctors educated
to examine that window, you demonstrated that we
are also sometimes privileged to reach through that
window and touch the soul that lives behind it.
Thanks for teaching me what eight years of
upper education could never teach.

*"The eye is the lamp of the body.
If your eyes are good,
your whole body
will be full of light."*

—Matthew 6:22

Acknowledgments

I am grateful and humbled by the number of people who have encouraged, facilitated, educated, and assisted me in writing this book.

To my wife, Janice, and our dear children, Michael, Jenna, and Mia: Thank you for supporting me and understanding why I needed it quieter in the house sometimes. I love you.

Scott Mactavish, thank you for walking me through the process and pointing me in the right direction. They say it's who you know. . . . I wish you the best in your continuing saga of success.

Michelle Goodwin and the doctors and staff of Primary Eyecare, thank you for being awesome. It is a blessing to be able to trust you all so much. Michelle, you are truly gifted—thanks for being my right hand in business.

Kristen Perkins, thanks for rolling with me as my hyper brain constantly causes your first priority of work to be an endlessly moving target. Your design work is brilliant and you have contributed significantly.

R. Bentley Calhoun, M.D., thank you for making time in your busy schedule to contribute to this book. Thank you for supporting our family—we are blessed to have you in our lives.

Mohit Nanda, M.D., a man of intelligence and surgical skill beyond belief, I thank you on behalf of our numerous mutual patients who you have single-handedly prevented from blindness. I am grateful for your scholarly review of my work.

David Cockrell, O.D., F.A.A.O., the walking dictionary and spreadsheet, I can't believe how you organize and file so much data in your brain! Thanks for being an advocate for optometry as well as supporting my book.

I am most grateful for the guidance provided by my publisher, Norman Goldfind of Basic Health Publications, Inc., during the development of this manuscript. John Anderson, thank you for applying your skillful talents while editing my work—you gave me a newfound appreciation for the craft and expertise required for the editing process. Gary Rosenberg, thank you for your considerable contribution of assembling this work and making it presentable—after all, a book about eyes needs to be "easy on the eyes." I would also like to express my gratitude to Mike Stromberg and Kristen Perkins for the artwork design they contributed to this work. I could not have completed this book without all of you.

Dad, you are my optometric and life hero. I question whether I would have made it through the first semester of college, let alone all the way through optometry school, without your encouragement and words of wisdom. You have my respect in so many ways.

Last but not least, I thank God for every blessing that He has graciously bestowed upon my life.

INTRODUCTION

Human knowledge to date has discovered quite a bit about how eyesight works, but we don't yet know everything. As much as we understand scientifically and neurologically, we still can't recreate eyesight in a laboratory (and I'm not certain that we ever will). We do know that there are things we can do to help enhance and protect our eye organs, to preserve them for as long as the rest of our body continues on.

Our eyes are a well-designed optical system, a complicated and highly developed organ. And we rely on them for just about everything we do in our lives, both personal and work-related. Eyes are the biological windows that allow us to behold the beauty of the world. The delightful gift of eyesight is one that we don't frequently stop to appreciate. A famous admonition reminds us to "stop and smell the roses," but when was the last time you considered what it would be like without the ability to see them too? It is an uncomfortable thought just to consider. Many cases and causes of blindness worldwide are entirely avoidable with proper health care. Just as a high-performance engine requires maintenance, tuning, and proper fuel balance to run smoothly, our eyes also demand the same. An improperly monitored and maintained engine (or eye) eventually operates inefficiently, runs poorly, or just shuts down entirely. That's why it is so important to take good care of our eyes.

A 2009 study conducted by the National Eye Institute found that the prevalence of nearsightedness, or myopia, rose by a whopping 66 percent in the United States since the 1970s. Forty-one percent of the United States population is estimated to have some degree of nearsightedness currently, an increase from 25 percent just three decades ago. Though the study did not investigate the causative factors, it is believed that the use of modern day technology such as computers, text messaging, cell phones, and smart phones may be contributing factors to the increased frequency of myopia. While the trend of life expectancy favorably continues to rise, it unfortunately brings with it higher incidences of age-related diseases: glaucoma, macular degeneration, and cataracts are all increasing in prevalence.

Like your physician, an eye doctor is a partner in health care. Unfortunately, many people have the misperception that being able to read the "20/20 line" on an eye chart is an indication that they don't need to have an eye examination. Just as "routine physicals" are known for effectively detecting early disease in an otherwise healthy person, an eye examination assesses the overall health of the eye, which entail much more than just reading letters on an eye chart. Often, a very diseased eye can still achieve 20/20 vision, leading the person to a false sense of security. Our eyes work tirelessly, but they ask little from us in return, with the exception of regular maintenance. Having vision examinations on a regular basis is the way to ensure that your eyes are providing the clearest and most comfortable vision they are capable of delivering. Just as important, regular comprehensive eye examinations monitor the health of the ocular tissues. For many people, an eye examination means not only precise vision, but the difference between life and death. Daily, people who otherwise thought they were just getting their eyeglasses updated during a "routine eye examination" are first diagnosed with serious, life-altering conditions. Diabetes, cancer, liver dysfunction, uncontrolled blood pressure, an impending stroke, brain tumors, and high cholesterol are all potentially discoverable during an eye examination. How much worse is the quality of life and prognosis when the discovery of these conditions is delayed or *never* made?

ALL IN THE FAMILY

My family has been involved in eye care for three consecutive generations. Jim Vincent, my father's uncle, began practice as an eye doctor in 1955. He was vital in helping direct my father's career path into eye care in the late 1960s. My father, "Dr. D," has been practicing optometry since 1975, and twenty-one years later I became an optometrist as well. Eye care is in the Di Girolamo family blood. I also married my optometry school classmate and sweetheart, Janice, so our family conversations involve a bit of eye care, too.

When I was only four years old, I attended my father's graduation from optometry school, and even at that young age I could appreciate the gravity of the occasion. I recall the pride I had telling my friends that my dad was an eye doctor. As an elementary school student, I was fascinated with the examination room instruments, eye charts, and lens grinding tools that my father had in his office. I shadowed him at work many days, sitting in during eye exams and watching the entire office operate as a team, resulting in a new pair of eyeglasses for the patients who needed them. By the time I was in sixth grade, I had a part-time job doing odds and ends around the office. My very first work assignment was filing charts—you would be correct in saying that I started at the bottom and worked my way up. I found out that work was difficult, not all glory and white lab coats.

Like thousands of other southern Californians, I had an eye exam performed by my dad each year. I recall having three or four consecutive years in which my vision tested at a perfect 20/20. Oddly, I was slightly disappointed about the good results because my father didn't get to "fix" anything on my eyes. However, at age eleven, the eye chart wasn't as sharp and distinct as it had been previously. My diagnosis was nearsightedness, and I was excited to see my dad go into action to solve my vision problem. While he led me out of the exam room, he said "Okay, we'll need to pick out a pair of eyeglasses for you now." Wait, I thought, eyeglasses? Other people may need to wear eyeglasses, but my dad is an eye doctor! I just wanted him to heal me of nearsightedness.

I have learned a thing or two since then.

THIS BOOK IN FOCUS

This book is organized to present eye health and vision maintenance in a logical and easy-to-use manner. Basic eye anatomy and tips for preventing vision problems are presented first. This is information that everyone should read. The remainder of the book then looks at specific eye problems.

A number of common vision abnormalities are covered in detail:

- Nearsightedness

- Farsightedness

- Astigmatism

- Presbyopia

- Light sensitivity and glare

- Poor night vision

- Computer vision syndrome

Eye problems that are associated with aging are presented to help you with vision correction for your entire family:

- Children—including conjunctivitis, amblyopia, color blindness, and nystagmus

- Adults—including dry eyes, glaucoma, and keratoconus

- Seniors—including cataracts and macular degeneration

A number of other factors may affect the health of your eyes, and these are covered as well:

- Injuries and infections

- Headaches

- Systemic diseases (diabetes, hypertension, high cholesterol, thyroid disease) and sexually transmitted diseases

Finally, I also provide an "insider's guide" to getting the best vision care for the dollars you spend.

A BIT OF CLARITY

My purpose in this book is to present reader-friendly information about how eyes function, their malfunctions, maintenance, and care. Eye doctors try to take the complex matters of ocular physiology, optics, and health and explain them to our patients in easy-to-understand ways. Unfortunately, in the name of efficiency and cost cutting, today's managed care environment means that many patients spend less time with their doctor. Even without this influence, an hour or two with your eye doctor would still be insufficient to cover the basics each of us should know about eye health. Patient education about diagnoses, causes, mechanisms, and preventative measures against future eye conditions is critical for vision care and maintenance. This book is not meant to replace your eye doctor but to clarify your understanding of eye health issues.

I look forward to sharing with you the fascination that I have with our beautifully complex and highly functioning sense of sight.

PART ONE

EYE CARE BASICS

CHAPTER 1

ANATOMY
OF THE EYE

*The only thing worse than being blind
is having sight but no vision.*
—HELEN KELLER

The human eye is a perfect model of a well-designed optical system. However, it is not absent of all flaws since many people need vision-correcting devices. Despite our tremendous knowledge of optical systems design, humans have not been able to surpass the eye's elaborate and beautiful design. The eye is a complicated and highly developed organ of magnificence. In the early embryonic stages of development, the eye originates as a direct neurological extension of the brain.

Today's cameras work well because they are modeled after the design of the human eye. The eye dynamically adapts to different light conditions and depths of field, various speeds of movement, and an infinite spectrum of colors. Modern cameras can accommodate most of these things well, too. Our eyes allow us to see in bright light conditions or in very dim illumination. We are able to focus on images only an inch away from the eye (at least when we're younger) or images at great distances. The required change in our eye's focus between the two distances happens in a fraction of a second, so rapidly that the brain can't even detect the lag

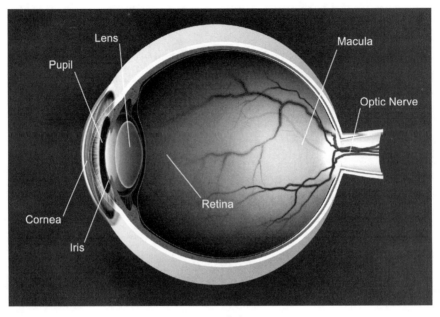

Anatomy of the Eye

between the two. The eyes provide us with depth perception, color differentiation, and peripheral and central vision. They truly are our window to the world.

Objects at various distances from the eye—and even a single object—have differing types of light rays that enter the eye. Take, for example, light rays entering the eye from a book held sixteen inches away versus light rays from the same book being held six feet away. The eyes need to process and focus the light rays at those two distances differently. Similar to a camera, the eye has multiple lenses that adjust the focus of light entering the eye depending on the distance of the object. In an eye that doesn't require eyeglasses, all of the incoming light rays are acted on by the eye's lenses to perfectly focus the images on the retina.

Depending on the ambient light conditions at any given moment, the iris instantaneously adjusts the aperture (the opening called the pupil) to allow just the right amount of light to enter the eye. In dim illumination, the pupil dilates (increases in diameter) to allow in more light, and in bright conditions it constricts (decreases in diameter) to block excess light. Once the light has passed through the eye's lenses and pupil, the retina's job is to receive, assimilate the input from each eye, and process the millions of light rays. It then shuttles the information to the brain via the optic nerve, the "highway" that transports the information to the occipital lobe of the brain. From there, visual information is processed and feedback is given. If the brain detects the eyes viewing a tiger running toward them, the brain then tells the rest of the body to get busy running in the opposite direction. If the eyes view a piece of chocolate cake, the brain tells the mouth to salivate and get the digestive enzymes ready to go.

We will now take a look at the individual components of our remarkable sense of sight.

CORNEA

The cornea is the clear, dome-shaped covering over the colored part of the eye. About the thickness of a fingernail, this transparent tissue is made up of five layers. It is a somewhat soft tissue that can change shape by direct pressure or by a tightly fitting contact lens. The cornea's role is to begin the bending (refracting) of light that enters the eye to properly focus it on the retina. The cornea is lubricated and partially nourished by the normal tear layer (not the tears of crying).

Contact lenses are placed on this part of the eye as well. Laser eye surgery reduces or eliminates blurry vision by reshaping the corneal tissue so that it will perfectly focus light on the retina. Eyeglasses, contact lenses, and eye surgery are all ways to improve vision from an imperfectly shaped cornea.

Though the cornea is clear, millions of pain receptor nerves reside here. A corneal abrasion or foreign body rubbing on the cornea can be unbelievably painful. I've observed seemingly small abrasions incapacitate the toughest of men. One woman compared her corneal abrasion to the pain of childbirth (although most women have told me "not quite"). All those pain receptors enable our body to tell us if something is wrong with the cornea. Fortunately, the cornea has an amazing ability to regenerate tissue quickly to repair any damage done to it.

IRIS

The colored part of each eye is the tissue called the iris. The pupil is the black "donut hole" in the center of the iris. On a microscopic level, the iris is a beautifully weaved and textured mesh of peaks and valleys. Like a louvered window shade, the amount of light entering the eye is regulated by the iris controlling the size of the pupil. More or less light is allowed into the eye by how wide (dilated) or narrow (constricted) the iris tissue becomes. Two muscles reside in the iris and act in opposition. One is a "sphincter" muscle that causes the iris to flatly stretch out and make the pupil smaller when light conditions are bright. The opposing muscle is a "radial" muscle. Anatomically, this radial muscle is spread out through the iris like the spokes of a round bicycle wheel. Under contraction, the radial muscle fibers cause the iris tissue to bunch up, similar to window drapes bunching up when fully opened. This enlarges the pupil, allowing more light to enter the eye in dim or dark illumination.

PUPIL

The pupil is not actually tissue but the hole that the iris creates in its center. It is the black circle that you see in the center of the eye. A dilated pupil has a larger diameter and a constricted pupil has a smaller diameter. The pupil diameter in a normal eye constantly adjusts to the variable light levels in the environment to optimize eyesight. Only when the ambient light levels remain constant does the pupil size remain the same.

LENS

Each of us is born with a naturally clear lens inside the eye, simply called the "physiological lens" or the "crystalline lens." About
the width of a pencil eraser, this lens further refracts (bends) light
after the light's passage through the cornea on the journey to its
ultimate destination, the retina. The physiological lens resides
directly behind the iris and is mostly covered by the iris. Not much
of the lens is visible to the naked eye of an observer. It is an adapt-
able and flexible clear tissue with the purpose of making "on the
fly" focusing adjustments to keep focused images on the retina.
The outside edges of the lens are attached to a muscle inside the
eye called the ciliary muscle, which exerts force to change the
shape of the lens. The ciliary muscle instantaneously alters our
focus by either contracting to put the lens under tension or by
relaxing to let the lens rest in its normal state. This process is
called *accommodation*. The pulling and releasing of the lens causes
the lens shape to change, allowing our eyes to focus on images at
different distances. Like manually focusing a camera by rotating
the lenses, this method of focusing happens due to the ciliary muscle tightening or releasing its grip on the lens.

Like our skin, the lens continually generates new cells as the
old ones die off. New skin cells push up from the deepest skin
layers as the outer, older skin cells die and flake off our body.
However, inside the eye, the lens does not have the same option of
flaking off old cells, since it has no place to discard the dead cells
internally. Instead, old lens cells are pushed inward toward the
center of the lens as the new cells generate from the outside-in.
Over many decades, this process of compacting cells inward
causes the lens to become less flexible when the ciliary muscle
attempts to act on it. This is the reason that most people around
age forty begin having trouble focusing on images up close. At this
age, the lens inside the eye can't readily adjust and focus as easily
as it once did.

RETINA

The retina is the neurological lining on the inside curvature of the eye. Like a miniature, bowl-shaped projector screen, the retina receives and maps the images our eyes are viewing. The purpose of the cornea and lens is to focus light onto the retina. The retina has numerous microscopic layers. Many people recall studying in school about the "rods and cones" of the retina. The rods are retinal cells that aid in the processing of low-light (night) vision, and the cones are the retinal cells that help process vision in normal light. The rods do not contribute to color vision, hence the inability to discern colors in dim illumination, and the cones provide the color vision we are accustomed to under normal lighting.

The retina is a complex tissue made up of intertwining nerves, cellular structural support systems, arteries, and veins. The information from the retina is collected and then "packaged" and sent to the brain for further processing. The optic nerve is the two-way "highway" that connects the retina and brain. Information carried via nerves, and oxygen carried through arteries and veins are all transported in and out of the retina via the optic nerve highway. Numerous bodily diseases can severely, and sometimes irreversibly, damage the retina, including diabetes, high blood pressure, and high cholesterol. Because the retina is so rich in blood supply, the functioning of the arteries and veins are critical. The eye itself can even have a "stroke" if the arteries and veins are not functioning normally.

MACULA

The macula, or fovea, is a specific, pinpoint area of the retina in each of our eyes and it corresponds to the very center of our vision. When you look directly at an object, it is the macula you're utilizing to see the object, and the remainder of the retina outside of the macula provides us with all of the less detailed vision around the object being viewed. The macula in each of our eyes has the densest concentration of cells in the entire retina. Using digital photography as an analogy, the macula has ten megapixels of resolution comparatively to the remainder of the retina, which has only three megapixels of resolution.

OPTIC NERVE

The optic nerves are the second pair of the twelve cranial nerves. Each of the optic nerves (one for each eye) is a large "super-nerve" comprised of millions of smaller nerves bundled together from the retina. The optic nerve is likened to a large telephone wire leaving a neighborhood; it is made up of many smaller cables bundled together from each individual home. As mentioned earlier, the optic nerve carries information in both directions between the eyes and the brain. The optic nerve communicates from the brain not only to the retina, but it also provides the impulses to the iris to dilate or constrict for light regulation, as well as signals to several of the external eye muscles that turn the eye's gaze in different directions.

That covers the basic components of the eye. As you can see, it is a highly complex system, beautifully designed but also susceptible to many malfunctions. I will cover these potential problems, and what can be done to alleviate them, in the remaining parts of this book. But first, I want to talk about a number of steps you can take to prevent vision problems and keep your eyes healthy.

CHAPTER 2

PREVENTATIVE EYE CARE

For decades, Americans have named vision loss as one of their greatest fears, second only to cancer. Some surveys have found that vision loss is even more feared than cancer. The National Eye Institute reports that 38 million Americans over the age of forty are blind, have severely reduced vision, or have an eye-related disease. Sadly, that number is on the rise. Vision loss and blindness take a significant toll beyond eyesight: the psychological impact of vision loss is colossal and, unfortunately, loss of sight has led countless people to suicide.

These grim reminders may help elevate the significance of taking steps now to prevent vision and ocular problems from manifesting later on. Though we are not able to remove the risk of all diseases just by good preventative care, we can significantly cut the risks of some diseases linked to certain habits and behaviors. Here, I list four "must do's" for preventing vision and eye problems.

"MUST DO" #1
GET AN EYE EXAMINATION REGULARLY

The first and easiest step in preventative eye care is to have a comprehensive vision and ocular health examination performed at least every one to two years. This is a critical activity whether you wear eyeglasses or not. Certainly having an eye examination takes time and money, but the return on investment is your eyesight! With modern diagnostic and treatment technology, many of the diseases and conditions in this book can be prevented or treated, but they must first be properly diagnosed.

Several major eye disorders create no obvious symptoms until they are too late to treat, so you may not be aware that you have a problem. Early detection and treatment are therefore critical to good ocular health and, potentially, to preventing vision loss. One study estimated that approximately 92,700 new cases of blindness each year would have been curable or preventable through timely detection and treatment.[1] Early glaucoma and early macular degeneration do not produce readily recognizable symptoms. However, the ocular signs of these diseases, along with examination instrumentation, allow the eye doctor to detect these threats early so that intervention may be instituted.

Seeing 20/20 on an eye chart is in no way an indication of *ocular* health, it is only an indication of *visual* health. Many people are lured into a false sense of security thinking that their eyes are healthy because they are able to read the 20/20 line on an eye chart during a vision screening. Though a visual acuity of 20/20 is a relative indicator of good ocular health, many visual disorders and blinding diseases can still be taking hold. These diseases are often well on the way to creating damage while an individual is still maintaining 20/20 vision.

The condition most notorious for this is glaucoma, a disease capable of causing irreversible blindness. Glaucoma is called "the sneak thief of sight," and nearly half of those who have it are completely unaware of it as they are slowly losing vision. Nearly 1 in 50 Americans has glaucoma, and approximately 1 out of every 100 people has glaucoma but doesn't know it. The risk factors for glaucoma are relatively easy for an eye doctor to detect during a comprehensive eye examination, even if you don't ask the doctor to specifically check for its presence. However, those risk factors won't otherwise be identified until it is too late to reverse damage.

Many people have been spared devastating visual loss because early signs of ocular disease found during a regular examination led to prompt medical intervention. Diabetes is a condition often first diagnosed through internal ocular manifestations. People with undetected diabetes may not have any unusual vision symptoms. Undiagnosed diabetics often go to the eye doctor simply to update their eyeglasses and the exam reveals diabetes. This is just one of the many systemic diseases that are first diagnosed during regular eye examinations each day across the United States.

With the widespread availability of eye care providers, isn't an eye examination at least every one or two years worth the investment? While the cost of an eye exam is a financial consideration, ask someone that has lost their eyesight what they'd willingly pay to have it back if they could. Even insurance companies recognize the importance of preventative care for the eyes and our health in general. Medicare covers eye examinations and glaucoma screenings for its members. Many other insurance plans also offer discounts and incentives for patients to participate in preventative health care programs.

Children should have their first eye examination performed by an eye doctor at 6 to 12 months of age. While pediatricians screen infants and children for vision problems, they admittedly catch only a small percentage of those who have ocular health needs. The pediatrician's screening is not a replacement for an examination with an eye doctor.

At the first examination, the eye doctor will make specific recommendations regarding the next examination interval. This recommendation will be customized to what conditions, if any, were diagnosed during the initial exam. See the charts on the following pages of the recommended eye examination intervals for children and adults according to the American Optometric Association (AOA).

The Two O's: Optometrists and Ophthalmologists

We lead busy lives and people usually think about eye care only once every year or two. The distinctions between optometrists and

RECOMMENDED EYE EXAMINATION FREQUENCY FOR CHILDREN

| | EXAMINATION INTERVAL | |
AGE	ASYMPTOMATIC/RISK FREE	AT RISK*
Birth to 24 months	At 6 months of age	By 6 months of age or as recommended
2 to 5 years	At 3 years of age	At 3 years of age or as recommended
6 to 18 years	Before first grade and every two years thereafter	Annually or as recommended

* Children considered to be at risk for the development of eye and vision problems may need additional testing or more frequent re-evaluation. Factors placing an infant, toddler, or child at significant risk for visual impairment include:

- Prematurity, low birth weight, oxygen at birth, grade III or IV intraventricular hemorrhage
- Family history of retinoblastoma, congenital cataracts, or metabolic or genetic disease
- Infection of mother during pregnancy (e.g., rubella, toxoplasmosis, venereal disease, herpes, cytomegalovirus, or AIDS)
- Difficult or assisted labor, which may be associated with fetal distress or low Apgar scores
- High refractive error
- Strabismus
- Anisometropia
- Known or suspected central nervous system dysfunction evidenced by developmental delay, cerebral palsy, dysmorphic features, seizures, or hydrocephalus

Reproduced with permission of the American Optometric Association (AOA).

ophthalmologists can be quite confusing. After all, eye doctors are found in a wide variety of locations such as medical complexes, shopping malls, surgical centers, department stores, strip malls, and hospitals. Let's begin by discussing the education and qualifications of each type of provider.

Optometrists—Optometrists are eye doctors who, after receiving

RECOMMENDED EYE EXAMINATION FREQUENCY FOR ADULTS

AGE	EXAMINATION INTERVAL	
	ASYMPTOMATIC/RISK FREE	AT RISK*
18 to 60 years	Every two years	Every 1–2 years or as recommended
61 and older	Annually	Annually or as recommended

* People at risk include those with diabetes, hypertension, or a family history of ocular disease (e.g., glaucoma, macular degeneration); people working in occupations that are highly demanding visually or eye hazardous; those taking prescription or nonprescription drugs with ocular side effects; people wearing contact lenses or who have had eye surgery; and anyone with other health concerns or conditions.

Reproduced with permission of the American Optometric Association (AOA).

a four-year undergraduate degree in pre-medicine, continue on for four more years of optometry school education, resulting in a Doctor of Optometry (O.D.) degree. Optometry school education, like medical school, begins after pre-medical undergraduate studies, where a degree in biology or chemistry is typically received. Optometry school concentrates on human and ocular anatomy, physiology, optics, refraction, pharmacology, and ocular disease management.

Among the many services they provide, optometrists are experts at optimizing the visual system of the eyes for the prescription of eyeglasses and contact lenses. Optometrists also diagnose, manage, and treat diseases, dysfunctions, infections, and chronic conditions of the eye. This includes the management of disorders such as cataracts, macular degeneration, and diabetic eye disease. Optometrists prescribe drugs to treat inflammation and diseases of the eye such as infections, glaucoma, dry eyes, conjunctivitis, and uveitis. Emergency services for the treatment of eye injuries, eye infections, and removal of foreign objects from the eye are common parts of an optometrist's responsibilities. If surgical intervention is required, optometrists will refer the patient to the appropriate specialist. The American Optometric Association estimates that approximately 38,000 licensed optometrists are practicing in the United States.

Ophthalmologists—Ophthalmologists are physicians and eye surgeons who, after receiving a four-year undergraduate degree in pre-medicine, continue on for four more years of medical school education, resulting in a Medical Doctor degree (M.D.) or Doctor of Osteopathy (D.O.) degree. Medical school education begins after pre-medical undergraduate studies, where a degree in biology or chemistry is typically received. After medical school, they continue residency training for at least another four years of specialized eye care and surgical training. Many ophthalmologists begin practicing "general ophthalmology" after their residency in ophthalmology. Most general ophthalmologists perform at least some surgical procedures, the most common type being cataract surgery. Like optometrists, general ophthalmologists examine patients to provide vision and ocular health exams for eyeglasses and contact lenses. They treat all eye infections and injuries, as well as chronic eye diseases such as glaucoma and macular degeneration. In addition to prescribing medications, ophthalmologists perform surgery as indicated in the treatment of ocular diseases.

Many ophthalmologists further specialize their education and surgical training beyond "general ophthalmology" to receive additional concentrated training in specific regions of the eye. Ophthalmology specialties include corneal and refractive surgery, cataract surgery, surgical and medical retina, neuro-ophthalmology, pediatric surgery, glaucoma surgery, and oculo-plastic surgery. Ophthalmologists who specialize in these areas frequently limit their practice to their specialty area to perfect their expertise and surgical skills. The American Board of Ophthalmology estimates that there are about 24,000 licensed ophthalmologists in the U.S.

Should I Choose an Optometrist or an Ophthalmologist?

Choosing an eye doctor is more confusing than it should be. The lines between the roles optometrists and ophthalmologists each play in the world of eye care are blurry. Decades ago, a sharp delineation separated which services optometry and ophthalmology practices each provided. Optometrists were known primarily for vision services (prescribing eyeglasses) and ophthalmologists were sought for disease management and surgical skills. However, today there is significant overlap between the services and care that optometrists and ophthalmologists each provide.

Over the last four decades, optometry has expanded beyond visual sciences and optics as its sole concentration of expertise. Contemporary optometry school education concentrates heavily on the diagnosis and treatment of eye disease. Much of what was considered the sole domain of ophthalmology forty years ago is now part of the regular scope and licensure of optometry. Ophthalmologists are still nearly the exclusive providers of ocular surgery. Ophthalmologists remain more medically oriented than optometrists, continuing to be the preferred professional for handling complicated ocular disease cases and surgery. Some ophthalmologists also provide eyewear and contact lenses in their practices, similar to optometry practices.

Optometrists are usually the first point of contact a patient makes in the eye-care system. Being cost effective and most accessible to patients, optometrists provide more than two-thirds of primary eye-care services. Because optometrists are frequently the first professional a patient seeks with problems concerning their eyes and vision, optometrists are trained to handle "most of the problems, most of the time." Just as a family physician refers patients to a specialist when necessary, optometrists recognize when specialized care is necessary for their patients. When indicated, optometrists will refer their patients to an ophthalmologist or other healthcare provider, who can best care for the situation if additional expertise is required. When surgery is required, or rare diagnoses and conditions mandate the expertise of a specialist, ophthalmologists are best positioned and trained to render the most specialized types of eye care.

It is useful to research the doctor's credentials and training,

DIFFERENCES BETWEEN OPTOMETRISTS AND OPHTHALMOLOGISTS

	OPTOMETRISTS	OPHTHALMOLOGISTS
Undergraduate education	4 years of pre-medical college; typically receives a degree in biology, chemistry, or psychology	4 years of pre-medical college; typically receives a degree in biology, chemistry, or psychology
Graduate school education	4 years of accredited optometry school	4 years of accredited medical school
Residency training	Optional	Yes
Surgical training	Limited but expanding	Yes
State licensing	Yes	Yes
Board certification	Optional	Optional
Performs ocular surgery	Limited: 12 U.S. states currently allow some surgery by optometrists.	Yes
Prescribes eyeglasses and contact lenses	Yes	Yes
Prescribes topical eyedrops	Yes	Yes
Prescribes oral medications, including narcotics	Yes	Yes
Areas of further specialization	Low vision Contact lenses Pediatrics Binocular vision Sports vision Vision therapy Rehabilitative services Computer vision syndrome Forensic optometry Limited types of surgery in some states	Cornea and anterior segment surgery Cataract surgery Glaucoma surgery Retinal disease/surgery Refractive laser surgery Neuro-ophthalmology Pediatrics/pediatric surgery Oculo-plastic surgery Oncology
Approximate number of practitioners in the U.S.	38,000	24,000

particularly when choosing a doctor to care for long-term conditions such as glaucoma and macular degeneration. Often, the best way to research doctors is through word-of-mouth reputation. Asking friends, neighbors, and co-workers about their experiences with local eye care providers is a great way to rapidly determine a consensus regarding service and expertise. A referral from a health-care professional is another way to find an eye doctor. You may also search online for optometrists at the American Optometric Association website (www.aoa.org) or the American Academy of Optometry website (www.aaopt.org), or for ophthalmologists at the American Academy of Ophthalmology website (www.aao.org). Starting in 2011, all health-care providers, including optometrists and ophthalmologists, will be ranked by governmental entities (Medicare) and by all major health-care insurers.

"MUST DO" #2
TAKE NUTRITIONAL SUPPLEMENTS

Everyone knows that proper nutrition is important for our bodies to function normally, and the eyes are no exception. Our bodies require specific nutrients to build healthy cells, to have proper nerve conductivity, and to provide the fuel to operate. It will likely come as no surprise that a diet rich in fruits and vegetables is most advantageous for the eyes.

Proper nutrition, and for some individuals nutritional supplementation, are important factors in reducing the risk of certain eye diseases, particularly macular degeneration and cataracts. It is important to assess your current dietary intake of vitamins and other nutrients, and weigh them against your risk factors for various eye diseases. This will help you to adjust your intake of vitamins and minerals in order to achieve optimal levels. Your primary care physician and eye doctor can help you assess whether you should utilize nutritional supplements.

Exercise and a healthy diet with abundant amounts of fruits and vegetables contribute to a higher quality lifestyle and a healthier body. Certain vitamins and nutrients are necessary for normal functioning of the eyes, as well as protection from various ocular diseases. Most people in the United States have access to a wide variety of foods in their diet. Consuming fruits and vegetables as part of a regular diet can provide all of the nutrients our bodies need. However, the individual diet of each person should be assessed for any deficiencies, and those deficiencies can then be compensated for with nutritional supplements. Though obtaining nutrients through the diet is preferred, supplements can serve to round out an incomplete diet.

Carrots are often the first vegetable that comes to mind when thinking about eye health. Carrots are rich in beta-carotene, which the body converts to vitamin A, and proper vitamin A levels are crucial to good eye health, regardless of age and disease risk factors. However, a common misperception is that a diet rich in carrots will keep vision "perfect" and prevent the need for corrective lenses. Unfortunately, carrots will not have any effect on the need for eyeglasses or contact lenses. Nevertheless, vitamin A is still crucial since it is a required nutrient to allow our night vision to function properly, as well as possibly providing protection against macular degeneration.

There has been strong interest recently in the use of nutritional supplements for eye health. However, solid, science-based studies with concrete evidence regarding supplements for eye health are few and far between. Much of what we understand today about ocular nutrition is still developing, but positive information is emerging. The pros and cons of vitamin supplementation should be considered on a case-by-case basis between patients and their doctors. Factors such as age, diet, family medical history, ocular history, medications, and current health status must be taken into account.

The Role of Vitamins in Ocular Health

Vitamins A, C, and E, zinc, and omega-3 fatty acids (fish oil) are all necessary nutrients for proper eye health. If you are not obtaining

Recommended Nutrients for Healthy Eyes

Did you know that daily intake of certain nutrients—either through foods or supplements—has been linked to healthy eyes and may reduce the risk of some chronic eye conditions?

Consider the list below, and remember that the recommended daily intake of these essential nutrients typically requires supplementation in addition to the amount consumed through traditional dietary sources. Ask your pharmacist or supplement retailer for details, and be sure to follow product directions. It is always important to consult your eye health professional or physician before beginning any new nutrition regimen, including when it changes your dietary supplement usage.

Lutein: 10 mg per day
Sources: Dark green leafy vegetables such as spinach, collards, or kale; corn; eggs; lutein supplements

DHA/EPA (Essential Fatty Acids): 500 mg per day
Sources: Flax, fleshy fish like tuna or salmon, fish oil supplements

Vitamin C: 500 mg per day
Sources: Orange juice, other citrus and fortified juices, citrus fruits, vitamin C supplements/multivitamins

Vitamin E: 400 IU per day
Sources: Nuts, salad and vegetable oils, peanut butter, fortified cereals, sweet potatoes, vitamin E supplements/multivitamins

Zinc: 40–80 mg per day*
Sources: Red meat, poultry, oysters, fortified cereals, nuts, baked beans, milk, multivitamin/mineral supplements

---

* The 40–80 mg zinc dosage is for people diagnosed as being at high risk for age-related macular degeneration (AMD) or experiencing early-stage AMD. The recommended dietary allowance (RDA) for zinc is 11 mg for men and 8 mg for women. High doses of zinc may cause stomach upset. Also, zinc supplementation has been known to interfere with copper absorption, so 2 mg per day of copper is strongly recommended for people supplementing their diet with zinc. Excellent sources of copper are mixed nuts, sunflower seeds, and beans.

Source: www.aoa.org

these from your diet, you may want to consider taking a daily multivitamin supplement, an ideal way of "filling in the gaps" of your diet to maintain a healthy body. The body excretes the excess vitamins through urination. Unless toxic levels of vitamins are consumed, or certain pre-existing conditions are present, over-the-counter multivitamin supplements are generally low risk. Multivitamin usage should always be discussed with your physician first, since they may cause problems in certain health conditions or when taken along with some prescription medications.

We have a good idea of what the ideal ocular supplements should be, but there has been only one solid, ten-year study researching this matter, called the Age-Related Eye Disease Study (AREDS). Completed in 2001, AREDS evaluated patients with various stages of macular degeneration and used a specific combination of nutrient supplements:

- Vitamin C (500 mg)   - Vitamin E (400 IU)
- Vitamin A (15 mg)   - Zinc (80 mg)

Patients in the study who followed the supplement protocol showed lower incidences and progression of macular degeneration compared to the control groups that received a placebo.

It is widely believed that the nutrients lutein, zeaxanthin, and omega-3 fatty acids may protect the macula and retina against damage from macular degeneration. However, these antioxidants were not evaluated in the original AREDS group. Strong evidence now exists that the nutrients possess protective factors, so many eye doctors are already recommending that their "at risk" patients use these supplements. A new study (AREDS II) is currently underway to assess the benefits of these nutrients. AREDS II is specifically evaluating the ocular benefits of lutein, zeaxanthin, and omega-3s in patients at risk for, and with existing, macular degeneration. AREDS II (2006–2012) is testing the following nutrients:

- Lutein (10 mg)

- Zeaxanthin (2 mg)

- Omega-3 fatty acids (1 gram, containing eicosapentaenoic acid [EPA] and docosahexaenoic acid [DHA])

The results of the study are anxiously awaited and should be available in 2013.

In some ocular conditions, particularly macular degeneration, larger doses of specific nutrients may have benefits in fighting the disease when it is already present. The original AREDS study showed that macular degeneration patients using the AREDS formulation achieved an approximately 25 percent reduced risk of developing catastrophic vision loss over a five-year period. There are several over-the-counter multivitamins that include the AREDS formulation, such as Bausch & Lomb's Ocuvite PreserVision Lutein and Alcon Laboratories ICaps. Several other companies also provide the AREDS formulation in their supplements.

Though supplements of lutein, zeaxanthin, and omega-3 fatty acids are certainly an option, they are also available in various foods:

Lutein: spinach, kale, corn, kiwi, pumpkin, zucchini squash, yellow squash, butternut squash, red grapes, green peas, cucumber, green bell pepper, and celery

Smokers and Beta-carotene

Beta-carotene supplementation is associated with a higher risk of lung cancer in cigarette smokers. *Cigarette smokers should not take beta-carotene supplements or the AREDS formulation supplements.* Research is being conducted about the risks for previous smokers taking beta-carotene but answers are still unclear, so beta-carotene is best avoided until further understanding is gained. Bausch & Lomb makes a formulation for smokers called PreserVision Soft Gels Lutein Eye Vitamins, which has no beta-carotene.

Zeaxanthin: spinach, kale, corn, orange bell pepper, oranges and orange juice, honeydew melon, and mango

Omega-3 fatty acids: salmon, cod, halibut, flax seeds, walnuts, and soybeans

"MUST DO" #3
PROTECT YOUR EYES FROM ULTRAVIOLET LIGHT

Ultraviolet (UV) light is a spectrum of light rays emitted by the sun and some electric arcs. UV light is subdivided into three ranges of wavelengths called UVA, UVB, and UVC. Most of the UV light emitted by the sun is blocked by the earth's atmosphere, but a small percentage (primarily UVA rays) passes through the atmosphere to reach the earth's surface. UV light can damage collagen tissues present in our skin and other body tissues, including the eyes.

Just as dermatologists recommend using sunscreen to protect our skin from damage caused by UV light, eye protection is also imperative. There are three specific, long-term ocular health concerns regarding chronic UV exposure to the eyes.

Pinguecula and pterygium: Pingueculas are the most commonly observed ocular tissue damage directly linked to excessive chronic UV exposure. A pinguecula is an overgrowth of tissue on the "whites" of the eye. They present as whitish-yellow raised areas at the 3 o'clock and 9 o'clock positions on either side of the cornea. People living in warmer climates closer to the equator receive more UV exposure than locations further north or south, so the prevalence of pingueculas in a given population corresponds well to their distance from the equator. Elevation also plays a role in UV exposure levels, with higher elevations receiving more UV rays. Though pingueculas are fairly common and are not sight threatening, they're known for becoming inflamed and irritated, a condition called pingueculitis. Pingueculas are often to blame for contact lens discomfort or intolerance.

If a pinguecula continues to be exposed to high levels of UV

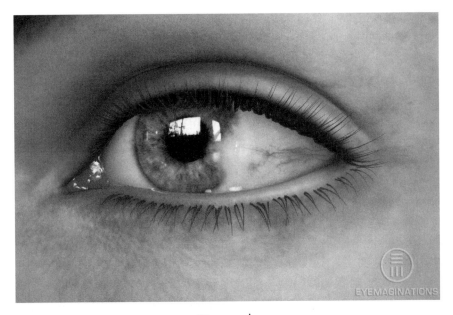

Pinguecula

light, it will grow larger in size and expand beyond the whites of the eye onto the clear cornea. A pinguecula converts to a pterygium when it crosses over the edge onto the cornea. As the wedge-shaped opaque growth makes its way toward the center of the cornea, it may affect the line of sight. A pterygium may eventually impede eyesight, potentially causing blindness. The opaque pterygium growth can be surgically removed, but often grows back over time, requiring multiple surgeries. Reducing or eliminating UV exposure to the eyes will help thwart the growth of existing pingueculas and pyerygia, or prevent their development in the first place.

Cataracts: Though a combination of multiple factors is believed to cause cataracts, UV light exposure appears to be a contributing factor. There is a high correlation between the age of onset of cataracts and environmental and lifestyle factors contributing to higher levels of lifetime UV exposure. For decades, UV light has been thought to be a main factor in the development of cataracts, but new research and data suggests that blue light in the visible spectrum may be more to blame than UV light. Either way, good quality sunglasses are imperative in protecting the eyes from both UV and blue light.

Macular degeneration: Like cataracts, macular degeneration has multiple contributing factors, but a chronically high level of UV exposure is one of the most highly correlated factors. Steps taken early in life to guard against excessive exposure to UV rays likely reduces the risk of this sight-threatening disease later in life.

One other health concern related to UV exposure is facial skin cancer. The eyelids are an area where skin cancers commonly occur. Because they are the body areas least protected from the sun, the face, eyelids, and arms are the most common areas for developing cancerous skin lesions due to UV exposure. Squamous cell and basal cell carcinomas are notorious for affecting the eyelid area. The judicious use of sunglasses, facial sunscreen, and wide-brimmed hats while in the sun are effective ways of reducing the damaging effects of UV light.

Recommendations

The most effective way of protecting the external and internal areas of the eye from UV damage is through the use of 100 percent UV blocking sunglasses and UV blocking prescription eyeglass lenses. Good quality non-prescription sunglasses, as well as prescription (clear ophthalmic and sunglass) lenses have the ability to protect the eyes from the majority of direct UV exposure. Be sure that the non-prescription sunglasses you purchase are marked as "100 percent UV blocking." Cheap, inferior quality sunglasses do not necessarily block all UV light, though they claim to be "UV blocking." In addition, choose larger sunglass lenses to protect a larger surface area of your face and eyes. A "wrap" style frame will best prevent light from entering from the sides compared to a smaller, non-wrapping frame style. Because some direct and reflected light rays may still reach the eye by passing through the gaps between the skin and the glasses, 100 percent UV protection to all areas of the eye is not possible without goggles. Nevertheless, the most dangerous direct UV rays are defeated by good quality sunglasses and eyeglasses.

Most plastic prescription eyeglass lenses today are treated with UV-400, the optical industry's standard product utilized to prevent the transmission of UV light through a lens. UV-400 treatment allows even clear (non-tinted) prescription lenses to block all UV light transmission. Make sure to ask if your prescription eyeglass lenses will block UV light. Polycarbonate plastic is a commonly used material for the fabrication of eyeglass lenses and it blocks UV light; no further UV-400 lens treatments need to be applied.

Many disposable contact lenses on the market today filter UV light and prevent most UV transmission into the eye. While this feature is desirable and helpful, it is not a substitute for wearing sunglasses. The UV filtering contact lenses do help to protect the internal eye, but they do not prevent UV exposure to the eyelids and some of the external eye tissues. Sunglasses will better protect the eyelids, so be sure to still use sunglasses even if you use UV-blocking contact lenses.

"MUST DO" #4
START A CESSATION PROGRAM IF YOU SMOKE

Everyone knows that smoking cigarettes is an unhealthy habit. Cigarettes rob the lungs of oxygen and replace it with lethal carbon monoxide. Besides the well-known association with lung cancer, emphysema, and cancers of the digestive system, cigarettes are harmful to the eyes as well. Unfortunately, the risk of developing almost any of the major ocular diseases covered in this book is much higher in smokers. Dry eyes, cataracts, macular degeneration, thyroid eye disease, and diabetic eye disease are all more common in smokers.

Tobacco fumes irritate and inflame the conjunctiva, the clear outer layer of the eye. Smokers typically have chronically bloodshot and irritated eyes. To make matters worse, cigarettes can cause dry eye along with the other associated annoying symptoms.

Among many conclusions that the large Physicians Health Study determined was a direct link between cigarette smoking and the incidence of cataracts.[2] As tobacco fumes become absorbed into the bloodstream, the destructive ingredients are delivered to multiple body systems, including the eyes. Several other studies have linked cigarette smoking with increased risks for diabetic retinopathy[3] and thyroid eye disease.[4]

Probably the most frightening association of cigarette smoking and ocular health is the link to macular degeneration. Smoking is the most preventable risk factor for developing macular degeneration. Additionally, studies (including AREDS) have shown beta-carotene supplements to be beneficial in protecting against macular degeneration in patients at high risk for the disease, yet smokers are advised not to take beta-carotene supplements because they may increase their risk of lung cancer. Therefore, smokers simultaneously increase their risk of macular degeneration and disqualify themselves from the benefits of beta-carotene.

Smoking Cessation Help

It is always easier said than done, but smokers are unsurprisingly warned to quit the habit. The strongly addictive nature of nicotine makes quitting a formidable challenge, though not an insurmountable one. Over-the-counter and prescription smoking cessation aids can increase the success rate and cut down on the cravings and withdrawal symptoms. Counseling and support groups are also helpful. Physicians are glad to help their patients find resources and guide them in the process.

Anecdotally, I have had several patients who smoke tell me, "I'm gonna die from something, it might as well be something I enjoy." Unfortunately, blindness caused by smoking can occur well before death. Yes, we will all die, but blindness can be prevented by kicking the habit. Please seek help and start a smoking cessation program now.

PART TWO

COMMON
VISION
PROBLEMS

CHAPTER 3

REFRACTIVE ERRORS OF THE EYE

The bending of light is referred to as refraction. Light travels at different rates of speed depending on the clear media that it is passing through, causing light to be bent (refracted) differently as it passes through each different medium. For instance, light passes through air faster than it does through water. An example of this is apparent when you look at a straw placed in a glass of water. The straw appears to have a "break" in it at the junction between the water and air because light is traveling at different speeds. Though the straw is not really broken, the way light is refracted makes it appear as if it were.

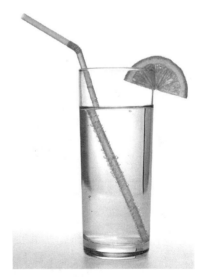

Glass and Straw

The eye is made up of several clear structures that light must traverse on its journey to the retina to be perceived as a clear image. To reach the retina, light must first pass through the air, the tear layer of the eye, the cornea, the aqueous fluid, the crystalline lens, and the vitreous fluid of the eye, with each structure contributing its own effect on the refraction of light. The cumulative refraction of light after passing through all of these structures ideally delivers the light in perfect focus onto the retina. If light is abnormally bent too much or not enough, the resulting image on the retina is blurry. When the eye's natural and unaided bending of light results in a blurry image, it is referred to as a "refractive error" of the eye. The purpose of eyeglasses, contact lenses, and laser eye surgery is to correct any error of refraction that interferes with the proper focusing of light onto the retina.

MYOPIA (NEARSIGHTEDNESS)

Myopia is the medical name for nearsightedness. Nearsightedness means that, without correction (eyeglasses and contact lenses), objects that are far away are more blurry than objects that are close up. With higher levels of nearsightedness, it can even be difficult to see objects that are very close as well. Similar to an

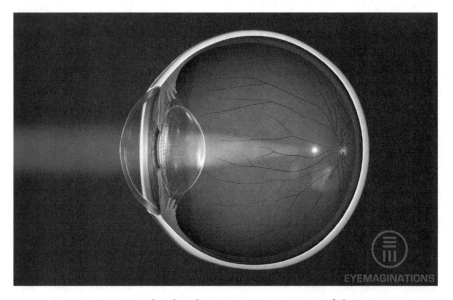

Myopia—Nearsighted Light Rays Focus in Front of the Retina.

out-of-focus projector that is too far away from the screen, myopia causes blurry vision because the light entering the eye is inappropriately focused prematurely in front of the retina.

Nearsightedness affects millions of people across all ages and nationalities. In particular, Asians have a very high incidence of nearsightedness. Some Asian countries have reported 70–90 percent of the adult population as nearsighted. Approximately 70 million American adults, or roughly one in four, is nearsighted. It is by far the most common refractive error.

What Causes Myopia?

The short answer is "no one is sure." However, it's thought that myopia is likely caused by a combination of hereditary and environmental factors. Myopia can be traced to heredity and its prevalence is often (but not always) higher in individuals whose mother and/or father were also nearsighted. However, no strong predictability pattern has been determined by geneticists. In many cases, children of two highly myopic parents never become nearsighted. Conversely, an individual may still become myopic even if neither parent was nearsighted. Experts disagree as to what level (if any) genetics plays in myopia, but a practiced eye doctor will likely tell you that their experience shows a genetic component.

External environmental factors such as excessive reading and computer use sometimes contribute to the development and progression of nearsightedness. Since I practice in a large university community, I observe this frequently. I have examined thousands of undergraduate and graduate students over my career, and nearsighted undergraduate students generally have a moderate increase in myopia during their college years compared to non-students. Other eye doctors and I have observed an even more dramatic rise in the incidence and progression of myopia among graduate-level students such as law and medical students. Normally, graduate students spend even more time reading than undergraduates and there appears to be a fairly direct correlation between the time spent on close work and the prevalence and progression of myopia. Various research studies have suggested that the prevalence of myopia increases in relation to the "intelligence" of the populations evaluated.

So, is nearsightedness genetic, environmental, or just dumb luck? Actually, it's probably a combination of all those things.

Levels of Nearsightedness

Nearsightedness is measured by units called diopters. A diopter is the measure of optical lens power, determined by the distance away from the lens surface that light is brought into perfect focus. A higher-powered lens has more diopters, and a lower-powered lens has fewer. A plus (+) diopter powered lens converges light together, causing it to focus earlier than without the lens. A negative (−) diopter powered lens diverges light and brings it into focus further away than without the lens. When looking at your eyeglass prescription, a minus sign (−) indicates a nearsighted prescription, which is then followed by numbers indicating the quantity of nearsightedness. A rough breakdown looks like this:

−0.25 to −3.00 diopters = mild nearsightedness

−3.25 to −6.00 diopters = moderate nearsightedness

−6.25 to −10.00 diopters = highly nearsighted

−10.25 diopters or higher = extreme nearsightedness

From an observer's standpoint, nearsighted eyeglass lenses (but not contact lenses) tend to minify the size appearance of the wearer's eyes in correlation to the strength of the prescription. Opticians are skilled at reducing this cosmetic effect with the proper selection of lens materials, lens manufacturing processes, and prescription-appropriate eyeglass frames.

Risks Associated with High Levels of Myopia

Higher levels of myopia (−6.00 diopters or more) are associated with an increased incidence of other ocular pathologies. The risk of these conditions typically increases as the severity of myopia increases. Your eye doctor can more specifically determine your individual risk after a thorough examination of your eyes.

Retinal Detachments: The greatest concern for a highly myopic individual is the increased risk of developing a retinal detachment. Overall, retinal detachments are infrequent, but they are more likely in someone with higher levels of nearsightedness. Anatomically, the length of the nearsighted eyeball is increased by up to a few millimeters compared to a normal eye. This additional eye length stretches the lining inside the eye (the retina). Just like pulling on both ends of a thin facial tissue, you can only stretch it so far before a tear develops. These same dynamics can occur in the eye. The retinal tissue inside a myopic eye is able to withstand some stretching, but it is under more tension as a result of the stretching. Depending on the level of retinal stretching, the retina may tear spontaneously or as the result of trauma to the eye.

The good news is that retinas at increased risk for detachment can often be identified ahead of time during a comprehensive ocular examination. Frequently, an eye doctor is able to identify areas of thinning or stress on the retina prior to a detachment. If the risk of a retinal detachment is severe, a surgeon may use a laser to "tack down" areas of the retina to reduce the risk. Most eye doctors strongly recommend that anyone with a myopic prescription of –6.00 or higher have a dilated ocular exam at least once a year to help identify this risk in advance. The adage "an ounce of prevention is worth a pound of cure" certainly applies here. (See Chapter 9 for more on the signs and symptoms of a detachment.)

Floaters: Floaters are a common occurrence in the eye, particularly as the eye matures. The development of floaters is facilitated in a myopic eye for the same reason that retinal detachments are more common—the length of the eye is once again to blame. A thick, clear fluid in the eye, called vitreous humor, is firmly attached at the back and also toward the very front of the eye. In between, the vitreous fluid is only loosely attached. The attachment at the front of the eye is stronger than the one at the back, so stretching of the eye in myopia sometimes causes the attachment at the back of the eye to become loose. This is called a vitreous detachment. After the vitreous humor detaches, it usually leaves distortions and aberrations in the vitreous fluid causing "noise" in the fluid, often referred to as floaters. Provided that there are not also flashes of light occurring in the eye, floaters are pretty harmless, but they can be extremely disturbing and frustrating. Though there is no cure or treatment, floaters often become less noticeable and bothersome over many years for most people. Floaters vary in size and shape from a minimal, barely visible floater to a large, prominent floater that never seems to go away.

Decreased Best Corrected Vision: Although 20/20 vision is considered a normal level of acuity for most eyes, not all "normal" eyes see 20/20 vision, even with correction. Some eyes see better than 20/20 and others don't see 20/20 perfectly, though they are still "normal." When the level of nearsightedness reaches –10.00 diopters or more, it is not unusual to find the eye incapable of reaching the 20/20 level of acuity even with eyeglasses or contact lenses. As prescriptions reach these higher levels of nearsightedness, acuities of 20/25 or 20/30 are sometimes the best result to be expected. In my experience, however, this rarely disturbs the highly myopic patient since their overall vision with correction is such a vast improvement over what they see without correction.

Glaucoma: Though the reasons are not fully understood, highly myopic individuals are two to three times more likely to develop glaucoma than someone without nearsightedness. Eye doctors check for signs of glaucoma during a comprehensive examination.

Controlling Nearsightedness

There are no surefire ways of eliminating nearsightedness, with the exception of laser eye surgery, and even that is not completely guaranteed. However, there are steps that can be taken to help control the progression of myopia, techniques that will help some individuals but not all. Because myopia has so many contributing factors, these techniques are not guaranteed either, but no harm is done in trying them, and many people feel they have been helped by them.

A Separate Prescription for Reading:
Using Multifocal Lenses or Reading Glasses

For decades, many eye doctors have recommended a separate pair of reading glasses or a multifocal-type lens for rapidly progressing nearsighted individuals. Because of the additional costs associated with it, this separate "reading prescription" method is not routinely prescribed in the treatment of myopia but is reserved for cases when the patient or parent is very concerned about the myopic progression and desires to intercede.

Nearsighted prescriptions usually change most rapidly from ages 7 to 18. It is thought that lengthy reading (or any type of near work) puts too much stress on the eye's natural focusing system and induces myopia to progress faster by a gradual lengthening of the eye. Instead of focusing by the eye's natural method of accommodation, the reading glass prescription allows the ciliary muscle to relax while still providing clear vision. Eye doctors will normally suggest this option when the myopic prescription is changing rapidly every 3–6 months, or when the discussion is brought up by a concerned parent of a child with rapidly progressing myopia, asking "Is there *anything* that we can do?"

It is difficult to quantify the exact beneficial effect that reading glasses may have because we don't know what the individual's prescription would have been if they weren't using them. Nevertheless, this approach still has significant merit. Patients with a steady and predictable rate of myopic progression over time (for example, a –1.00 diopter change every six months for the last two years) will usually observe a slowing in the rate of progression after initially using reading glasses. Doctors regularly observe this as well and may offer a reading prescription as an option to consider. My preferred method of discussing this topic with patients is educational in nature, similar to what I've described here. We know nearsightedness is multifactorial—genetics and environment play a role. The only potential negative of this option is the added expense of an additional pair of eyeglasses or multifocal lenses. If the additional cost factor were removed, I'd likely recommend this for all of my young, progressively myopic patients, though it is not always guaranteed to work.

A small study on this topic that was undertaken several years ago provided somewhat mixed results. The Correction of Myopia Evaluation Trial (COMET) studied 469 children and the results of the study after three years showed that progressive additional lenses slowed myopia progression in the children by a small, but statistically significant, amount. However, at the five-year mark (COMET 2 Study), it was reported that the study subjects showed similar rates of nearsighted progression regardless of using multifocal or single-vision lenses.[5]

I advise you to work with your eye doctor to choose the best option for your particular prescription, needs, and lifestyle.

Rigid Gas Permeable Contact Lenses

Conventional rigid gas permeable contact lenses (RGPs) may also play a role in myopia control. Both the lengthening of the eye and the increasing curvature of the cornea are factors that occur in progressive myopia. Rigid gas permeable lenses may be able to address the increased steepening of the cornea over time. RGPs can have a retainer-like effect on the cornea, since the cornea's soft tissue conforms itself to the shape of the back surface of the lens when worn on a regular basis. Some of the desired retainer effect wears off once the RGPs are discontinued, but we surmise that there is some residual improvement. As with the reading glasses option, it is difficult to prove what the progressively worsening prescription would have been if the RGPs weren't used. However, in patients with rapid, predictable patterns of myopia progression,

RGPs interrupt that trend and sometimes slow it down permanently. Speak with your eye doctor regarding your particular rate of progressive myopia to discuss if this is an option you should consider. If you are going to wear contact lenses anyway, this might be a reason to choose rigid gas permeable lenses instead of a soft contact lens. There are pluses and minuses to each type of contact lens that extend beyond this "retainer effect," so you should consider this in lens selection.

Ortho-Keratology (Ortho-K) builds on the inherent molding effect of rigid gas permeable lenses and takes it to a further degree than just holding the cornea in place. With Ortho-K, highly customized RGPs are used to gently reshape the cornea to the exact curvature that produces no nearsightedness or astigmatism. Ortho-K allows some nearsighted and astigmatism patients the benefit of 20/20 (or sometimes better) vision. The lenses are worn overnight while sleeping to allow the cornea to take on the shape of the contact lens. When the lenses are removed upon awakening, the temporarily induced shape of the cornea provides clear vision, without the use of contact lenses or eyeglasses. This reshaping effect stays in place for 24–48 hours without re-inserting the contact lenses again.

Ortho-K contact lenses were used by some eye doctors as early as the 1970s, but the rudimentary manufacturing of the lenses at the time limited the prescription ranges and success rates. Today, the technology and safety of wearing these lenses overnight has improved to the point that, in 2002, the U.S. Food and Drug Administration (FDA) approved a lens made by Paragon Sciences (www.ParagonCRT.com) for this purpose. Paragon's lens is called the Corneal Refractive Therapy (CRT) lens and is approved for treating up to –6.00 diopters of nearsightedness and up to –1.75 diopters of astigmatism. Bausch & Lomb also received FDA approval for a proprietary Ortho-K lens called the Vision Shaping Treatment (VST) lens. Eye doctors are required to receive additional manufacturer training and certification before fitting patients in the lenses.

Generally, patients with lower amounts of nearsightedness and astigmatism achieve the most favorable results from Ortho-K. The benefit that CRT and VST lenses have over laser surgery is that the induced corneal changes are reversible. If at any time you want to go back to your original prescription, the cornea will return to its original curvature a few days after you stop wearing the lenses. With regular follow-up visits to the eye doctor, these lenses are safe for overnight use when worn and cared for as prescribed. Ortho-K lenses need to be replaced on a regular basis (approximately once a year) to preserve proper amounts of oxygen transmission through the lenses. These overnight lenses carry the same slightly increased risk of infection as conventional overnight contact lenses. It is critical that you adhere to your doctor's instructions and maintain a recommended follow-up schedule.

Frequently Asked Questions About Myopia

Will wearing eyeglasses make my nearsightedness worse?

This question comes up frequently. If you are over twenty-five years old, most often the answer to this question is no, wearing eyeglasses is not contributing to your myopia. However, if you are younger than twenty-five, there is a possibility in some environments that your eyeglasses may contribute to the myopic progression. It's plausible that using eyeglasses for extended periods of near vision (reading, computer), when your nearsightedness is not bad enough to warrant their use up close, may contribute to progression over time. If your nearsightedness is less than –2.50 diopters, you can still read clearly without correction. My recommendation is to remove your eyeglasses when reading if you are able to still comfortably see. In a classroom situation where frequent changes in focal distance occur (looking back and forth between the front of the class and your notes), it is not practical to put the glasses on and take them off each time the focal distance changes. However, with sustained reading or computer work, it is advised to remove the glasses. Not wearing a

Dispelling the Myths

William Bates, M.D. (1860–1931), was an ophthalmologist who developed what is known today as the "Bates Method," an alternative health program of vision improvement. He asserted that refractive errors such as nearsightedness and astigmatism were directly caused by stress on the eye, and they could be improved naturally without eyeglasses. However, many of the claims that he made about the eye are based on flawed physiological assumptions. The Bates Method employs techniques such as "palming" and "sunning." Palming is the process of covering one's eyes (without pressure) so that all light is prevented from entering them. Dr. Bates asserted that in the total absence of light, the eyes are allowed to de-stress and relax, paving the way to better eyesight, but there are no scientifically proven cases of improved refractive error as a result of this practice. Sunning was a method of gradually training the eyes to tolerate and accept intensely bright light. When fully trained, the student of sunning supposedly could stare directly at the sun without consequence other than improved eyesight, according to Dr. Bates' 1920 book *Better Eyesight*. It is well known today that this is not only an ineffective practice but, more important, an unsafe one. Staring directly at the sun is known to physically burn the sensitive retinal tissue in the eye called the macula (solar maculopathy).

Additionally, the Bates Method includes an eye exercise program to aid in the natural improvement of nearsightedness and farsightedness. In his book *The Cure of Imperfect Sight by Treatment without Glasses*, Dr. Bates states, "It has been demonstrated in thousands of cases that all abnormal action of the external muscles of the eyeball is accompanied by a strain or effort to see, and that with the relief of this strain the action of the muscles become normal and all errors of refraction disappear." Today, it is known that the external eye muscles do not play a role in focusing light inside the eye. The external eye muscles move one's gaze in different directions rather than acting in a focusing capacity. It is the ciliary muscle *inside* the eye that plays a role in focusing light (refraction), yet the exercises advocated by Dr. Bates did not affect the ciliary muscle. Anyone who has had their eyes dilated likely recalls the subsequent blurry vision, which occurs as a result of the temporary disabling of the ciliary muscle. The same dilating eyedrops do not affect the external eye muscles, which Dr. Bates claimed to play a role in focusing. Thus, other factors beside external eye muscles contribute to the clarity of our vision.

Alternative therapies to eyeglasses and contact lenses such as the Bates Method have enjoyed persistent awareness over the last several decades because of their appealing message. In 1998, the American Academy of Ophthalmology (AAO) undertook a study of various treatment therapies to establish an official opinion of them based on scientific evidence. Most of Dr. Bates' claims of effectiveness were based on anecdotal testimonials, not scientific evidence. The AAO concluded that "no evidence was found that visual training has any effect on the progression of myopia. No evidence was found that visual training improves visual function for patients with hyperopia or astigmatism. No evidence was found that visual training improves vision lost through disease processes such as age-related macular degeneration, glaucoma, or diabetic retinopathy."

To this day, many types of natural vision improvement books exist and enjoy brisk sales. "Improve your eyesight naturally in 30 days," "Throw away your glasses forever," and other such claims make for an enticing message, but these methods have not been repeatedly or scientifically proven effective.

nearsighted prescription for distance viewing will not strengthen the eye. When wearing contact lenses, you may find it impractical to repeatedly insert and remove them. Instead, try putting reading glasses on over the contacts to counteract their effect, or simply remove the contacts when reading for long periods.

Is it normal for my vision to seem "weird" or to have headaches when I put on a new pair of eyeglasses?

Often, it takes the eyes and the brain a few hours up to a day or two to adjust to a new lens prescription. Any number of visual effects may temporarily occur, including a "swimmy" feeling, a barrel-effect to vision (where objects appear to bow out toward you), and an odd feeling of depth perception. In some cases, a mild or severe headache may also occur. Not only does the new prescription sometimes contribute to this, but the lens material, as well as a lens measurement called the "base curve," may require adaptation. Normally, these effects subside quickly and the new eyeglasses then feel great. However, if any of these effects last more than twenty-four hours, notify your optician about what you are experiencing. He or she will guide you through the adjustment period and also explain the contributing factors. In rare cases, the symptoms persist and the eyes don't adapt, requiring the optician (and sometimes the doctor) to resolve the source of the problem. For this reason alone, it may be wise to consider purchasing your eyewear from the same location as your doctor.

HYPEROPIA (FARSIGHTEDNESS)

Hyperopia is the medical name for farsightedness. Farsighted individuals not wearing eyeglasses typically complain of blurry vision or eyestrain up close but have clear vision when viewing objects far away. However, highly farsighted individuals find it difficult to see objects far away, too. Similar to an out-of-focus projector that is too close to the screen, hyperopia causes blurry vision because the light entering the eye has still not reached its focus by the time it meets the retina.

Hyperopia is separate from presbyopia, the age-related onset of blurry vision up close. Though the symptoms of farsightedness and presbyopia can often be the same, their causes are different. In fact, one may have both farsightedness and presbyopia simultaneously (see Chapter 4).

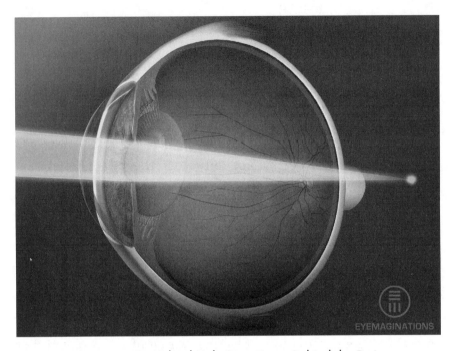

Hyperopia—Farsighted Light Rays Focus Behind the Retina.

The eye has a natural ability to compensate on its own for low amounts of farsightedness, unlike the inherent inability to do so in nearsightedness. With normal eye health, the eye is still required to "dial-in" a little correction for farsightedness by using its own ability when we read (see the section on the anatomy of the lens in Chapter 1). This "dialing-in" occurs only when we are viewing objects up close, but the brain knows to call on this same focusing mechanism to overcome mild amounts of farsightedness. The eye compensates for low amounts of farsightedness and often the individual is not symptomatic or aware that they are mildly hyperopic. As the levels of hyperopia increase, the eye will still compensate somewhat, but symptoms develop—individuals complain not so much of blurry vision, but of fatigue and headaches subsequent to short periods of reading and computer work. A pair of eyeglasses can relax the eyes and usually elicits an "ah, that just feels better" response from the individual.

Symptoms of higher levels of farsightedness mimic the same symptoms as nearsightedness. Sufferers of either extreme complain of blurry vision far away *and* up close. To further complicate and blur images, astigmatism may exacerbate the blurry vision at all distances. Your eye doctor can determine which of the conditions (or a combination) is causing the problem.

Levels of Farsightedness

Farsightedness is also measured by units of diopters. When looking at your eyeglass prescription, a plus sign (+) indicates a farsighted prescription, which is then followed by numbers indicating the quantity of hyperopia. The general categories of hyperopia are as follows:

+0.25 to +1.00 diopters = mild farsightedness

+1.25 to +4.00 diopters = moderate farsightedness

+4.25 to +8.00 diopters = highly farsighted

+8.00 diopters or higher = extreme farsightedness

From an observer's standpoint, farsighted eyeglass lenses (but not contact lenses) tend to magnify the appearance of the wearer's eyes somewhat. Opticians can mitigate this effect with the proper selection of lens materials, lens manufacturing processes, and prescription-appropriate frames.

Risks Associated with High Levels of Hyperopia

Fortunately, farsightedness is not associated with as many ocular health risks as nearsightedness. The primary ocular concern with hyperopia is "narrow angles," a condition in which more fluid is produced than is drained away in the eye. Under normal circumstances, the "faucet" inside the eye produces fluid at the same rate that the "drain" removes the old fluid. The purpose of this fluid production is to help maintain pressure in the eye and to carry nutrients to various parts of the eye. Farsighted individuals are anatomically predisposed to having a smaller drain that removes the fluid. If the drain is blocked or too anatomically narrow, the internal eye pressure can increase as excess fluid builds up, and this may subsequently lead to glaucoma if it goes undetected. During a comprehensive exam, the drainage mechanism is evaluated by the eye doctor, regardless of your prescription. If there is concern that the drain may not be functioning properly, the doctor may perform a further examination of the drainage mechanism in a procedure called gonioscopy.

Controlling Farsightedness

Unfortunately, there are no known methods of slowing down or reversing farsightedness other than the conventional methods of eyeglasses, contact lenses, or laser vision correction. Though reading glasses are often needed to correct for low levels of farsightedness, their use has not been shown to affect the progression rates of farsightedness.

ASTIGMATISM

Astigmatism is a refractive error like nearsightedness and farsightedness. It is not a disease; rather, it is a distinct vision problem causing blurry vision, often blurring focal distances both far away and up close. Astigmatism usually exists in combination with myopia, hyperopia, and/or presbyopia.

Light rays travel in all directions—light enters our eyes in vertical and horizontal directions, as well as every diagonal direction in between. With astigmatism, each direction of light focuses on the retina with a different prescription. Take the example of the letter *T*. Light (images) from the vertical and horizontal components of the *T* enter the eye at the same time. The vertical part of the *T* and the horizontal part each have different prescriptions for the eye with astigmatism. For example, the vertical component of the *T* may have a prescription of –3.00 while the horizontal component has a prescription of –5.00. The diagonal light in between the

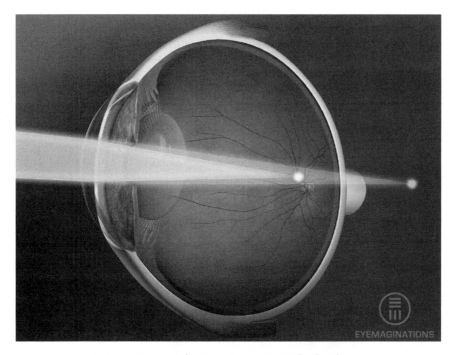

Astigmatism—Light Rays Focus in Multiple Planes.

vertical and horizontal is a prescription of somewhere between –3.00 and –5.00, depending on how close the light ray direction is to the vertical (–3.00) or horizontal (–5.00) components of the *T*. With high levels of astigmatism, a large disparity exists between the two prescriptions, and with low astigmatism, the values are much closer to each other.

Astigmatism blurs eyesight at all distances, both near and far. Patients with moderate or high levels of astigmatism typically report their vision to be blurry when they are reading, while working on a computer, *and* when looking at distant objects.

While lower amounts of astigmatism may not cause everyone to have symptoms when looking into the distance like higher levels of astigmatism do, lengthy near work such as computer viewing or cross-stitching may cause those even with very low amounts of astigmatism to complain of eye fatigue, blurriness, and fluctuating vision. Nearly two-thirds of people requiring eyeglasses have some astigmatism component to their prescription, so it is more common to have astigmatism than not. Like myopia and hyperopia, it is normal for astigmatism to fluctuate somewhat from one eye exam to the next.

Levels of Astigmatism

Like nearsightedness and farsightedness, astigmatism is measured by units of diopters. When looking at an eyeglass prescription, a minus sign (–) or a plus sign (+) in the "cylinder" box of the written prescription indicates an astigmatism prescription, which is then followed by numbers indicating the location of astigmatism, also known as the axis. A rough breakdown looks like this:

0.25 to 0.75 diopters = mild astigmatism

1.00 to 2.50 diopters = moderate astigmatism

2.75 to 4.75 diopters = high astigmatism

5.00 diopters or higher = extreme astigmatism

Your prescription will also indicate the affected eye(s):

O.D. = Latin abbreviation for right eye

O.S. = Latin abbreviation for left eye

O.U. = Latin abbreviation for right and left eyes together

Though each eye has only one prescription, optometrists and ophthalmologists often record eyeglass prescriptions a little differently. Optometrists normally write eyeglass prescriptions using "minus cylinder," which means the cylinder (astigmatism) component is recorded with a minus sign. Ophthalmologists typically write eyeglass prescriptions in "plus cylinder," meaning that the astigmatism component is recorded with a plus sign. But don't worry, your eyeglass lenses will be made correctly using either method.

R̸ EYEGLASS	SPHERE	CYL	AXIS	ADD	PRISM
R	-3.25	-0.50	130	+2.25	
L	-2.75	-0.75	082	+2.25	

DATE _____

PATIENT NAME _____ PATIENT # _____

REMARKS _____

_____

EXP. DATE _____ _____ . O.D.

Spectacle Rx

Controlling Astigmatism

Like nearsightedness, astigmatism may be slowed or controlled somewhat by external factors. There are no definitive ways of eliminating astigmatism, with the exception of laser eye surgery, and surgery is not completely guaranteed either. However, many of the steps that can be taken to help control the progression of myopia may also be effective with astigmatism, since astigmatism can be considered an optical variation of nearsightedness. In my experience, the most effective (but not guaranteed) methods of slowing or reducing astigmatism are the daily use of conventional rigid gas permeable lenses, or the more customized version of rigid gas permeable lenses called Ortho-Keratology. RGPs often temporarily improve astigmatism levels by flattening the cornea. Though difficult to prove, RGPs may also possibly contribute to the stabilization of astigmatism by deterring the cornea from further steepening over time.

CHAPTER 4

PRESBYOPIA

Middle age brings about many changes. At around age forty, most people begin to notice their eyes' inability to focus well on objects close to them (presbyopia). Regardless of whether you've worn eyeglasses previous to your forties or not, presbyopia affects virtually everyone. Early symptoms include having to hold reading material further away, blurry vision up close in dim illumination, inability to distinguish fine details, and eyestrain/fatigue toward the end of the day. Most people discover on their own that moving something farther away from their eyes aids the ability to see near objects during early presbyopia.

Just as our sense of hearing declines with time, so does our ability to see up close. The ability of our eye's internal lens to focus on near images diminishes with maturity. The lens no longer shifts the focus from far to near effortlessly as it once did. The word *presbyopia* comes from Greek and Latin origins that mean "old eyes." I've never dared to tell patients that they have "old eyes"! Rather, I explain that the blurriness is simply "a part of the maturing pro - cess." Generally that comment produces a smile and a look of terror at the same time. The first thing that usually pops into their heads is the "B word"—bifocals. Not everyone needs bifocals, however.

Prior to age forty, our eyes normally focus up close by involuntarily flexing the ciliary muscle inside each eye. Since the ciliary muscle is directly attached to the lens, the flexing and relaxing of the muscle changes the shape and focus. As we mature, the muscle still functions well, but the lens gradually loses the flexibility it once had. This loss of lens flexibility is what prevents our eyes from focusing properly up close as we age. I'm frequently asked by patients if eye exercises will help strengthen the eye's ability to read after the onset of presbyopia. Unfortunately, eye exercises do not improve this condition because the root cause is not muscular in nature—it's the loss of lens flexibility. Many false claims have been made in books and television infomercials about reversing this condition naturally or through exercises without the need for reading glasses. I wish it were possible to reverse this process without vision-correcting devices, but it simply can't be done.

Periodically, patients will claim some relative of theirs lived to 95 years old and never needed reading glasses. While these cases are probably true, there are usually valid explanations for it that are left out of the story. For example, if a person is nearsighted,

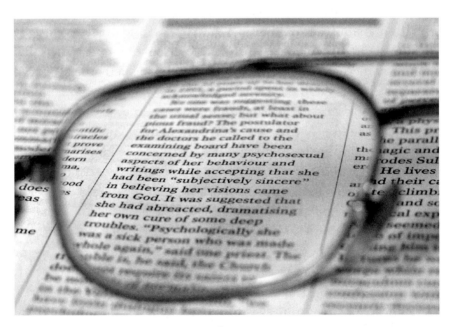

Presbyopia

they can read well without glasses, but they don't see clearly in the distance. They then live with the distance blurriness and claim, "I don't need eyeglasses." Another explanation is that the individual reads little or not at all. Finally, some individuals really do see moderately well far away and up close without eyeglasses. If only one eye has just the right amount of nearsightedness and the other eye has none, the nearsighted eye sees well up close without glasses. This leaves the other eye to see well in the distance. Occasionally, nature allows that little "prescription blessing" in an individual and they truly see well both near and at a distance without vision correction.

The exact age of onset for presbyopia varies from person to person and is mainly dependent on what type of eyeglass prescription (if any) they've had prior to presbyopia. A "normally" sighted individual who has never worn eyeglasses typically begins to notice symptoms of presbyopia around forty to forty-one years of age. A nearsighted individual, however, usually doesn't experience presbyopic symptoms until a few years later. In most circumstances, the more nearsighted someone is, the longer they go before complaining of near vision problems related to presbyopia. Nearsighted individuals normally experience symptoms anywhere from ages forty-two to fifty. This is myopia's one silver lining— nearsightedness forestalls the onset of symptoms caused by presbyopia. On the other hand, farsighted individuals may begin experiencing presbyopic symptoms as early as their late thirties.

Presbyopic patients regain their ability to see up close by various means. The most common way is the use of reading glasses. If an individual required an eyeglass prescription before the onset of presbyopia, that person will now have two, and sometimes three different prescriptions with the onset of presbyopia.

The type of visual work performed and the environment are two external factors affecting both the onset and severity of symptoms caused by presbyopia. A data entry processor who spends eight hours a day in front of a computer or an attorney who spends his or her day reading finely printed documents will suffer more symptoms earlier and more severely. A truck driver or a farmer, for example, usually won't put as much demand on their eyes from near work during the day. By evening when they try to read the newspaper, their eyes struggle less because they don't suffer fatigue from reading all day. Also, working in an environment that is bright allows our eyes to focus with less effort than in a poorly lit environment. Restaurants with dimmer "mood" lighting make reading a menu more difficult.

MANAGING PRESBYOPIA

There are a number of different solutions to presbyopia:

- Reading glasses
- Multifocal eyeglasses
- Monovision
- Multifocal contact lenses
- Laser vision correction
- Combinations of eyeglasses and contact lenses

Most people start with the simplest solution—reading glasses—at first. As people visually (and psychologically) become more comfortable with the idea of reading glasses, they often progress to the more individualized solutions discussed further below.

Reading Glasses

The natural lens inside the adult eye can "dial in" +2.50 diopters or more of focusing power prior to the onset of presbyopia. In newborns and children, the natural lens is capable of accommodating for up to 3–4 times that amount of power. The process of the eye changing power on its own is called "accommodation," and from the time we are born, we gradually lose the ability to accommodate. Our eyes need about +1.00 diopter of power over our regular distance prescription (if there is one) to focus clearly at a distance of 20–22 inches away—a typical distance that a computer monitor is from our eyes. A book is normally held about sixteen inches from the eyes, requiring up to +2.50 diopters of focusing.

The closer the object is to our eyes, the more accommodation they need. Presbyopia is the reduction and eventual absence of the eyes' self-accommodating ability. It is not until approximately age sixty that the eye has zero remaining ability to accommodate. Between ages forty and sixty, reading is accomplished by a combination of the eyes' remaining accommodative ability and a reading prescription.

So, if we need +2.50 diopters to read at sixteen inches from our eyes, and at age fifty the eye can still accommodate approximately +0.50 diopters without help, then adding +2.00 reading glasses gives us the focus we need. The reading glass power that we need over our distance prescription is fairly predictable by age.

READING GLASSES BY AGE

Age	Power Needed (Estimate)	Age	Power Needed (Estimate)
40–42	+1.25 diopters	50–54	+2.00 diopters
43–45	+1.50 diopters	55–59	+2.25 diopters
46–49	+1.75 diopters	60+	+2.50 diopters

The simplest solution for near vision problems is a pair of reading glasses. While reading glasses make our eyesight clear up close, they make our distance vision (further than six feet) blurry. Typically, a person who wears reading glasses will need to remove the glasses or at least look over the top of the lenses to see clearly in the distance. Since there are two prescriptions now, one for distance and one for near, reading glasses alone will help only the near distance as they simultaneously blur the distance. This is the method that most people adopt when they first begin to display symptoms of presbyopia. Single-lens reading glasses can be used if you don't need eyeglasses to see objects far away, either because you don't have a distance prescription or because you are already using contact lenses to make the distance clear.

Over-the-counter (OTC) reading glasses and prescription reading glasses each have pros and cons. OTC reading glasses (commonly called "readers," "magnifiers," or "cheaters") are inexpensive and don't typically require an eye examination or prescription to obtain. Most people use a "trial-and-error" method in the drugstore to determine their prescription. They try several pairs of readers until they find a pair that makes the reading distance clear. The inexpensive nature of these glasses, typically $10–$25 per pair, makes it easy to have multiple pairs of eyeglasses in several locations around home and at work. Using OTC reading glasses will not cause long-term harm to the eyes, even if you use a totally incorrect power. However, OTC readers have several drawbacks. The saying "you get what you pay for" certainly applies here. Over-the-counter lenses are "punched" out of inferior plastic and inserted in a cheap frame. Similar to a toy pair of binoculars, the optical clarity of the plastic lenses used is of poor quality, which inherently causes optical aberrations not present in an ophthalmic-quality lens. Other optical distortions or discomfort can be induced by an improper pupillary distance—each person has a unique distance between their eyes and this is accounted for in an ophthalmic pair of eyeglasses but only "averaged" in an OTC pair.

Another problem with OTC readers is that they only approximate your prescription. They are close but not exact for most people. Typically, people have some difference in prescription between the left and right eye even if they don't wear glasses for distance vision. Many also have mild astigmatism, which is not always critical to correct in distance vision, but is necessary for clarity and comfort close up. If you rely on your eyes to perform any substantial computer work or reading, OTC reading glasses are a poor choice. Briefly using a pair of OTC readers to read a recipe or pay a few bills shouldn't present much of a problem, though. OTC readers can also be handy in places you may not want to keep or use nicer eyewear, such as when fishing or in a workshop (use good safety eyewear over them, though).

OVER-THE-COUNTER VS. PRESCRIPTION READING GLASSES

OVER-THE-COUNTER READING GLASSES

Pros

- Inexpensive
- Less concern if broken or lost
- Available without a prescription
- Can be bought immediately off the shelf

Cons

- Less accurate; may induce eyestrain and fatigue
- Less comfortable fitting frame, "one size fits all"
- Break easily, have to be replaced frequently
- Unable to account for pupillary distance, may cause eyestrain
- Unable to account for different prescriptions in left and right eyes
- Cheap, misfitting glasses create a poor social impression
- Frames not easily adjustable

PRESCRIPTION READING GLASSES

Pros

- Better vision, visual comfort, and efficiency from exact prescription
- Easily adjustable frame and nosepads for proper fit
- Enhance your appearance; do not detract
- Account for pupillary distance measurement; better visual comfort
- Account for differences in left and right eye prescriptions
- Account for mild prescription components (e.g., astigmatism)

Cons

- More expensive
- Probably have fewer pairs lying around because of cost
- Not ready to be bought off the shelf, must be manufactured

Some contact lens wearers use OTC readers for near work. Any amount of astigmatism and differing prescriptions between the eyes can be accounted for by the contact lenses, which removes some of the problems with OTC readers. I recommend a high-quality pair of OTC readers if you and your doctor decide to go that route. Good "ophthalmic" quality ready-made readers are available at eye care providers for $50–$60.

Multifocal Eyeglasses

The most common and natural way of seeing well with multiple prescriptions for distance and near vision is through a multifocal eyeglass lens, which describes any type of lens that has more than one prescription in the same lens. The term *bifocal* means two prescriptions in the same lens, and *trifocal* means three prescriptions.

We've all seen lenses with horizontal lines in them. These are commonly referred to as "lined bifocals" or "lined trifocals." Benjamin Franklin is credited with designing the first bifocal lens by having his London optician cut his round eyeglass lenses in half and then glue the top half of his distance lenses to the bottom half of his reading glass lenses. When we read, our eyes naturally move to look lower and turn in toward our nose somewhat. This fact has made Franklin's bifocal lens design successful up through today.

However, today our measurements and methods of lens fabrication have evolved and improved quite a bit, and most individuals wear no-line bifocal lenses called "progressive lenses." Progressive lenses come in hundreds of designs and they get their name from the fact that the lens power becomes progressively stronger (for near) as our eyes look lower below the center of the lens. Progressive lenses cosmetically look nicer—they have no lines—and the lens looks the same as a single vision lens to everyone other than the user. Many people are anxious to hide the fact that their eyes are maturing.

Another progressive lens advantage is the way they work compared to a lined multifocal. From a functional standpoint, progressive lenses more closely mimic the way our eyes worked prior to needing a multifocal. There are no harsh lines that the eyes have to "jump" over as they move back and forth between the distance and near prescriptions. Rather, progressive lenses gradually transition power in the lens from distance to near, much like our eyes once did.

See the Appendix for further recommendations on selecting the right type of lens for your vision needs.

Monovision

Monovision is not a particular type of contact lens, but rather a different optical approach to getting clear images from the distance and close up. Monovision is the method of adjusting a person's contact lens or laser vision prescription to see clearly in the distance with one eye and clearly up close with the other eye. Typically, the dominant eye (the one you tend to prefer over the other) is the one chosen for the distance prescription.

Monovision is not without its drawbacks, though. A monovision prescription usually compromises depth perception. The Federal Aviation Administration (FAA) has banned pilots with a monovision prescription from flying commercial aircraft for this reason. Though monovision eyesight doesn't cause you to suddenly have such terrible depth perception that you immediately start rear-ending other cars while driving, many athletes complain of problems judging distances or reaction times when a ball is used in sports. Other complaints include difficulty navigating stairs or reaching to pick up a utensil.

As you might suspect, the clarity of vision is somewhat compromised with monovision. Our visual system is designed to function best when both eyes are focused on the same visual target. Monovision upsets this binocular functioning. In effect, monovision delivers only 50 percent of the visual information that our brain normally uses to process eyesight. In using only one eye to see far, the "near eye" is along for the ride since it is not contributing much to the brain's visual input. The eyes alternate their dominance at near, and again the brain receives only 50 percent of the visual input it normally has when reading, since only one eye sees well up close.

Monovision's artificially induced difference between the two eyes will not damage the eyes or visual system, but it throws the regular method of vision processing off track. It is far from a perfect solution to presbyopia, but it allows individuals the ability to achieve satisfactory vision without having to reach for reading glasses each time they look at their watch or write a check at the store. Though it has some drawbacks, I have numerous patients who have happily used monovision for twenty years and are still going strong.

The eye doctor evaluates each individual's lifestyle, visual needs, and prescription to help determine if monovision is a viable option. It is easy for the individual trying monovision for the first time to be a little discouraged at the initial visual result. Allowing the brain and the visual system to adapt to this new method of seeing can take up to ten days. Over that adaptation period, vision gradually becomes clearer and has a more natural feel. People often return a week or two after their initial monovision fitting and report that their vision seems much better. However, in a small number of people, adaptation never occurs, and monovision turns out to be a poor option. It is difficult to say in advance whether an individual will succeed or not with monovision. Trial periods of a week or two, as well as fine-tuning follow-up adjustments to the prescription by the doctor, are needed to really know.

With the development of better technology in contact lenses, fewer people opt for monovision as their first method of addressing presbyopia. More people are finding that multifocal contact lenses provide clearer and more comfortable vision than monovision, and multifocal contacts allow depth perception to remain unaffected.

Multifocal Contact Lenses

Multifocal contact lenses have improved through significant advances in technology in the last ten years or so. Though still not a perfect technology, today's multifocal contact lenses are a viable option for most people, depending on their visual needs. As you might guess, multifocal contacts are more complicated in design and manufacturing and they require much higher levels of professional expertise to fit and hone the prescription.

Many people initially assume, incorrectly, that multifocal contact lenses work like multifocal eyeglasses, where vision in the top half of the lens is for distance and the lower half of the lens is for reading. Though there are a small number of contact lenses that work this way, most multifocal contacts allow us to see using a totally different system of optics. The majority of multifocal rigid gas permeable and soft contact lenses utilize *aspheric* optical design. With an aspheric lens, the curvature of the contact lens differs in all areas of the lens, therefore creating various prescriptions in the same lens. One of the most popular designs used today relies on concentric rings of power in the contact lens.

Most multifocal contact lenses work by allowing the eyes to receive both the distance and near images at the same time. The brain effectively sorts out and processes these different images. Over the course of the first week of multifocal contact lens use, the brain learns to selectively "tune in" and "tune out" distance and near images as required. This sounds odd and complicated, but we know that our brains can handle complicated tasks. However, if we think about it, we also know our sense of hearing to function in quite the same way. Imagine having a conversation with someone at a cocktail party. Many other simultaneous conversations are occurring as the other guests socialize. Suddenly, you overhear someone near you in another conversation mention your name. Your hearing has the ability to "tune in" to that conversation and hear what is being said while your brain "ignores" the other conversations going on around you. You can then voluntarily "deselect" that conversation and switch to another, if desired, though the overall volume of the room never fluctuates much. Vision with multifocal contact lenses works the same way, and this visual process requires very little effort of conscious attention after the first few days of lens wear.

Vision with a multifocal contact lens is rarely described as "perfect" but rather it is more frequently described as acceptable or good. Many people use multifocal contact lenses because they will do anything to break free from the need for reading glasses for mundane tasks, such as writing a check at the store, checking email, and looking at their watch. For most people and prescriptions, these types of activities and seeing well in the distance are achievable with optimally fit multifocal contact lenses. Some higher-level prescriptions may preclude an individual from using multifocal contact lenses. Today, a few companies even make multifocal contact lenses that correct for astigmatism as well, and this recent development has opened the door to contact lens use for even more people.

My approach in counseling a potential patient before trying multifocal contact lenses is one of preparing them to have lower visual expectations. I explain to existing single-vision contact lens wearers that their distance contact lenses now give them perfectly clear vision far away, but zero clear vision close up (without reading glasses). A multifocal contact lens will potentially decrease the clarity in the distance they experience now to perhaps 90 percent (or greater), but in return it gives them 90 percent clarity at near, where they have none now. For most people this is acceptable, but certain individuals or visual tasks are incompatible with less than absolute clarity.

The type of work that the eyes are asked to perform is critical to the success of multifocal contact lenses. Someone who spends a great deal of time on a computer or reading (two hours or more continuously) will generally be unsatisfied with the vision provided by multifocal contact lenses. However, some people accommodate for various visual demands by switching between multifocal contact lenses and another vision correction method like reading glasses when the circumstances demand clearer vision than the multifocal contacts provide.

Combinations of Eyeglasses and Contact Lenses

A successful and commonly used solution to presbyopia is wearing contact lenses to correct only the distance vision (approximately six feet away and further) and then putting on a pair of reading glasses over the contact lenses to provide clear vision close up. The benefits of this combination are very clear vision/optics, reasonable costs, and ease of use. There is no "adaptation" period for this option, unlike with multifocal eyeglasses, multifocal contact lenses, and monovision, which do require adjustment.

The main drawback of combining contact lenses and eyeglasses is that it is often inconvenient. Reading glasses need to be carried along everywhere that you may need to see up close. If you forget to bring your reading glasses, there won't be much chance of seeing anything up close. Using this option, you'll frequently put the eyeglasses on and take them off as needed, and many people regularly take off their reading glasses and then forget where they've left them. It can be a hassle reaching for reading glasses every time you want to look at your watch, flip through the mail, or write a check at the grocery store.

Laser Vision Correction

"What about that laser surgery, will it help me?" This is one of the more frequently asked questions from my patients. Laser surgery is a viable option for many people, but only a doctor is going to be able to advise you accurately, after a thorough examination, if you are a good candidate.

If you are nearsighted, an option you may consider is monovision LASIK laser eye surgery (see more information on LASIK surgery in the Appendix). The laser eye surgeon can design your post-surgical prescription similar to monovision contact lenses, so it results in clear distance vision in one eye and clear near vision in the other eye. If you have not previously worn monovision contact lenses, the doctor will fit you in contacts before the surgery to allow for adaptation and to verify that you will be happy with the visual results. A monovision contact lens prescription is easily reversible if you are not happy; monovision laser surgery is not as easily reversed, though it's not impossible.

Conductive keratoplasty (CK), approved for use by the U.S. Food and Drug Administration (FDA) in 2002, is a refractive surgery procedure for farsighted individuals. CK creates the opposite effect on the cornea that LASIK does: LASIK surgery flattens the cornea to eliminate nearsightedness, whereas CK steepens the cornea to help eliminate farsightedness. CK can also be used to create a monovision method of eyesight, and it provides slightly better distance vision than the same monovision prescription achieved by contact lenses.

During the CK procedure (which is normally done in office), the surgeon gently taps a probe that emits radio waves to the outer edges of the anesthetized cornea. It is a painless procedure (at worst, patients sometimes complain of a gentle sensation of pressure on the eye). The radio waves cause the collagen tissue to tighten up. As the collagen fibers tighten in the peripheral cornea, the cornea bows more steeply in the center. Unfortunately, the steepening effect of CK is not permanent, and in most cases the initial effect regresses to the pre-surgical prescription after a few years. CK can be performed multiple times, though, provided that you don't mind paying for it again.

CHAPTER 5

Light Sensitivity, Glare, Poor Night Vision, and Computer Vision Syndrome

LIGHT SENSITIVITY

Light sensitivity (photophobia) has many causes that can be broken down into two main categories: natural or external. The uncommon but sometimes serious medical causes of light sensitivity, including meningitis, are not fully covered here. A recent onset of light sensitivity warrants a visit with your eye doctor.

Natural Causes of Light Sensitivity

Large Pupils

The pupil is the black at the center of each eye (actually an opening) that allows light to enter. Our pupils dynamically adapt to the amount of light around us, regulating the amount of light that enters the eyes. Each person's natural pupil size is slightly different than everyone else's. People with anatomically larger pupils take more light into the eye, just as a larger window transmits more light than a smaller one. Individuals with larger physiological pupils are often naturally more sensitive to light simply for this reason.

Light-Colored Eyes/Fair Skin

Melanin is the pigment that gives our skin its complexion. It also functions to absorb light; therefore a person with a darker complexion doesn't burn in the sun as easily as a fair-skinned person does. The same process applies to the eyes. People with blue eyes have the least amount of melanin in their eyes, and people with dark brown eyes have the most. Lighter-eyed people are more light sensitive because they have less ocular pigment to absorb the incoming light, whereas a brown-eyed person has ample pigment to help absorb light. Albinism is a condition where there is a total lack of body pigment. People with albinism suffer with severe light sensitivity because there is no ocular pigment to help absorb light entering the eyes.

Migraines

Migraine sufferers often have symptoms of extreme light sensitivity during their migraine event. Migraines frequently cause both photophobia and hyperacusia (an increased sensitivity to sounds), and any type of light or sound stimulus is completely overwhelming and painful during a migraine for many people. Thus, a dark and silent room is the most comfortable place to be for someone suffering from a migraine. Fortunately, these symptoms subside once the migraine is gone. (See Chapter 11 for more information.)

External Causes of Light Sensitivity

Medications

Numerous medications include "increased light sensitivity" somewhere in their long list of possible side effects. When a patient complains of a recent onset of light sensitivity, the first question a doctor usually asks them is, "What drugs are you currently taking, and have you started taking any of them recently?" Medications are one of the major causes of light sensitivity. The same nervous system pathways responsible for controlling pupil size are acted on by some prescription medications. As the nervous system is altered by these drugs, the pupil may become larger, allowing additional light into the eyes. Examine the possible side effects of any medications you use, particularly any new ones recently added, to determine if light sensitivity is a side effect. It is still important to notify your prescribing doctor of your symptoms even if you're relatively certain the light sensitivity is from a medication.

Some common medications known to cause light sensitivity include:

- Tetracycline
- Doxycycline
- Atropine
- Amphetamines
- Cocaine
- Idoxuridine

- Phenylephrine
- Scopolomine (motion sickness drugs)
- Trifluridine
- Vidarabine
- Eyedrops used by a doctor to purposely dilate the eyes

Dry Eyes, Eye Infections, Keratitis, and Contact Lens–Related Ocular Inflammation

When the cornea (the clear dome over the colored part of the eye) is compromised or stressed for any reason, an inflammatory response typically occurs. Just like a bee sting causes pain, swelling, and tenderness in the localized area, a similar inflammatory response occurs within the cornea when it is under stress. When fluid build-up (edema) and inflammation of the cornea occur, light entering the cornea is abnormally scattered and can cause extreme photophobia. Light sensitivity caused by infection or inflammation typically subsides once the underlying cause is resolved.

A Solution for Photophobia

One simple solution to light sensitivity is reducing the amount of light that enters the eyes. Dimming or turning off indoor lights, closing window shades, and wearing sunglasses (especially polarized lenses), are all great ways of controlling the discomfort stemming from light sensitivity.

GLARE

Glare is different than light sensitivity. Stray light rays entering the eyes reduce the overall contrast that our eyes are accustomed to having. Contrast is the discrimination between multiple colors and shades to define where one image ends and the other begins. On a white piece of paper, black print has more contrast than grey print.

Types of Glare

Bright Environments

Glare can exist anywhere there is bright light. Drivers have all experienced glare while driving into the sun at sunrise or sunset. The intensity of the sunlight low on the horizon affects the contrast of everything else that the driver sees. Environments that are naturally bright often further induce glare when a source of reflected light is present. Water and snow are two causes of intense glare on a sunny day. Under bright sunlight, our eyes already receive abundant light, and added to that is the extra light reflected off the snow or water. Glare can be a problem indoors, too: actors on

Glare

stage under theater lights experience glare from the intense amount of light focused on them; the high-intensity lights of a warehouse frequently cause glare.

Though more awkward indoors, the best way to control glare is to use polarized sunglasses. Polarized lenses filter out some of the stray light rays by allowing only rays of a certain direction to pass through. This counteracts glare by filtering out horizontally oriented light rays and reducing the overall amount of light entering the eyes.

Computer-Related Glare

Computer monitors are notorious for creating glare. Like environmental glare, computer glare is related to the volume of light entering the eyes. Glare induced by monitors is a cause of eye fatigue and discomfort for millions of people around the world every day. Computer monitors are self-illuminated and the monitor surface has mirror-like properties that cause light external to the monitor to be reflected off the screen. Subsequently, the eyes receive light from multiple sources.

A handy test can quickly reduce computer glare. Turn off the power to your computer monitor and take note of what reflections are still seen on the screen. See a reflection of fluorescent lights overhead, or a window from behind? If so, your monitor is causing glare. Sometimes simply tilting the monitor or turning a window shade will help eliminate glare from the monitor. In some cases, people have asked their maintenance department at work to remove the fluorescent lights from the fixture directly above their cubicles at work to reduce glare. If those options don't exist, a high-quality glare-reducing filter for your computer screen will help. A quality filtering screen can be an investment of several hundred dollars; I personally recommend the 3M brand of computer glare filters. It has been my experience that poor-quality glare reduction filters are just as bad as not having any filter. Some employers may help pay for the glare filter when the employee's eye doctor has recommended it.

Glare While Driving

While driving, we are susceptible to many sources of glare: from light reflected off the windshields of other cars, from wet roads, from reflective highway signs at night, and from street lights and traffic signals. Driving is a minefield of glare!

Daytime glare is significantly improved by using polarized sunglasses, which are available in prescription and non-prescription form. Polarized lenses even help on cloudy days. To reduce both daytime and nighttime glare, non-glare lens treatments (often called "anti-reflective" lenses) for prescription and non-prescription lenses help tremendously (see the Appendix for more information). While special lens tints (often yellow) are suggested for night driving to reduce glare, I do not recommend anything that reduces the amount of light reaching the eyes while driving at night. Do not wear sunglasses when driving at night, even if they reduce glare, because the negatives of driving at night with sunglasses outweigh the benefits they have on glare.

There are several techniques to safely reduce glare while driving at night without compromising your vision:

- Adjust side mirrors so that headlights from behind aren't directly reflecting into the eyes.

- Likewise, adjust the rearview mirror to the "nighttime tilt" for further glare reduction. Some automobiles today do this automatically.

- Make sure *both* sides of the windshield are perfectly clean—I can't overemphasize this enough. Make sure the windshield washer fluid is topped-off and use it as frequently as necessary to keep the windshield unobstructed. Also, replace the windshield wiper blades regularly so that they don't streak and further contribute to glare. Bugs, debris, dust, and dirt all act to scatter light rays that are entering through the windshield.

- Make sure to clean the inside of the windshield glass frequently. Often, vapors from solutions used to clean interior vinyl and leather fog the inside of windshields over time. Interior window surfaces of convertibles are susceptible to becoming dirtier than those of a hardtop. Fingerprints on either side of the glass don't help either.

- Have a mechanic check the alignment of the headlights. If the headlight beams are aimed too high or too low, vision will suffer. Other drivers on the road will also be negatively affected if the headlights are out of alignment.

Glare Caused by Poor Optics

Regardless of environment, glare is often caused by poor or damaged eyeglass lenses. Scratched lenses are one of the main causes of glare. Old eyeglass lenses that have not been cared for properly can "delaminate" and older treatments applied to the lenses using technology outdated by today's standards cause peeling and flaking of the lens surface. "Photo-chromic" lenses that automatically get darker outdoors sometimes develop a yellowish discoloration after many years. Chips, scratches, pits, and markings on eyeglass lenses all contribute to the scattering of light and increased glare. Inspect your eyeglasses for these issues, or have your eye doctor or optician inspect them and point out any clarity-reducing flaws. Even if your prescription hasn't changed, you will still experience improved vision and decreased glare if your lenses are replaced regularly.

Though soft contact lenses don't suffer from scratching like eyeglass lenses, rigid gas permeable contacts (RGPs) can scratch as they age and may be a significant contributing factor to glare. If your RGP lenses are more than four to five years old, there's a good chance they have some scratching. Unlike eyeglasses, scratches in RGP lenses can sometimes be polished away. However, if the lenses are five years old, they are likely due to be replaced for other reasons (like warpage).

It may be obvious, but having the most current and accurate prescription in your eyeglasses and contact lenses also reduces glare. Astigmatism is a particularly large contributing factor to glare and visual haloes. Glare is often the main complaint an individual reports when their astigmatism prescription has changed. Don't underestimate the big improvements in glare reduction that can be made with "small" changes in your prescription.

Cataracts

Cataracts are likely the single largest underlying cause of glare. However, someone suffering from glare doesn't necessarily have cataracts. A cataract is a cloudy opacification of the normally clear lens inside the eye. The cloudy cataract lens scatters incoming light and converts what would have been clear light rays into glare.

Cataracts reduce the volume of light just as a filter would, and how much filtering occurs depends on the density of the cataract. Cataracts bring on a vicious cycle of glare. A person suffering from cataracts requires more light than normal to see in order to overcome the decreased light volume reaching their retina. Unfortunately, as illumination is increased to compensate for the cataract, light scattering and glare increase too.

Prior to having a cataract surgically removed, the main options that exist to help reduce glare are polarized sunglasses and a non-glare ("anti-reflective") lens treatment for eyeglasses. Many people are familiar with the large shield-type sunglasses that have a sizeable surface area on the front, as well as the large side area that fully blocks sunlight. Though from a cosmetic standpoint they aren't very attractive, they are very functional. The large surface areas on all sides, along with the edges that curve toward the face, are very effective at blocking the stray light rays responsible for glare. Conventional sunglasses work well too, but some of the glare-causing light can still make its way into the eyes from the sides, underneath, and above conventional sunglass lenses.

Glare Caused by Ocular Inflammation

Temporary causes of glare and light sensitivity often originate from various forms of ocular inflammation. These can include the following:

- Corneal abrasions

- Contact lens–related eye inflammation

- Changes in the retina from diabetes

- Foreign bodies in the eye

- Conjunctivitis (pink eye)

- Dry eyes

- Burns of the eye (for example, from welding, UV light)

- Iritis or uveitis (ocular pain caused by inflammation of the iris or uvea, an internal covering surrounding the globe, which can happen in isolation or secondary to another systemic disease, typically autoimmune disease)

Edema, swelling secondary to fluid build-up, is part of the body's normal inflammatory process, whether stemming from a wound, an allergic reaction, or even an eye infection. Fluid related to inflammation can accumulate in the cornea, which is normally a clear tissue. The retina is also susceptible to fluid build-up. While fluid migration to parts of the eye that are injured or inflamed is helpful in the healing process, it can scatter light while it's there. The "healing" fluid temporarily interrupts the normal tissue functions that allow us to see, and introduces "noise" into the optical system. Fortunately, this temporary side effect subsides once the inflammation calms down and the underlying cause is removed. When glare is caused by inflammation, sunglasses (even used indoors) can be very effective at making you more comfortable.

POOR NIGHT VISION

It is common to experience blurrier vision at night than in the day, even if our vision during the day is normal. The lower levels of light available at night give our eyes less data to process. Several factors may contribute to abnormally poor night vision, and often only an eye doctor can diagnose the root cause after a thorough examination. However, there are some things for which to be on the lookout.

At night, the eyes naturally experience night myopia: because of the reduced light available, our eyes struggle to find a fixed distance or point to focus on, and they will assume a default focal distance. This default mode can cause the eyes to be nearsighted temporarily, even if they aren't nearsighted under regular circumstances. Night myopia can be so bothersome to some individuals that they wear eyeglasses at nighttime only.

Whether eyeglasses are worn regularly or not, a slight change to the prescription is often initially revealed by a reduced ability to see well at night. Minor shifts in the prescription are often too subtle to notice during the day, but these minor changes often become larger shifts at night. When the slight shift in the prescription is added to the already present night myopia effect, the cumulative change becomes visually significant. Often, the solution to this is simply updating the prescription to eyeglasses or contact lenses. This can be just a slight change of –0.25 diopters to the nearsighted or astigmatism components of the prescription, but it may involve a more sizeable shift.

Glare is frequently a source of poor night vision, too. Scratched eyeglass lenses, cataracts, and dirty windshields all contribute to reduced night vision. For a thorough discussion of how to reduce glare, see the previous section.

Other, less frequent but more serious underlying causes may also be the source of poor vision at night. People who have previously undergone refractive surgery such as LASIK or PRK may be left with a reduction in night vision, though technically they still read 20/20 or better on the eye chart. With today's modern laser technology, this side effect is less of a concern, but still a small possibility when undergoing refractive surgery.

Diabetes is a known cause of reduced clarity of vision at night.

The eyes are one of the main organ systems affected by diabetes, which can cause areas of swelling or bleeding inside the eye. Usually, these signs develop in direct relation to two things: the time that diabetes has been present and the highest level that the uncontrolled elevated blood sugars reach. Diabetics without the ocular signs of diabetes should have their eyes examined and dilated a minimum of once a year, and more frequently if they have been previously diagnosed with diabetic eye changes. Controlling blood sugar levels helps reduce night vision problems related to diabetes, and your eye doctor and primary physician will guide you through this process.

One of the most serious causes of significant night vision problems is thankfully somewhat rare. Retinitis pigmentosa is a group of ocular genetic disorders. Several variations exist and they each have a different inheritance pattern. This condition is frequently diagnosed in childhood. Night vision is significantly impacted in retinitis pigmentosa, even to the point that little or no vision exists at night. This night blindness is usually far more devastating than just reduced vision at night, which generally prompts an appointment with an eye doctor.

Retinitis pigmentosa is relatively easy for an eye doctor to recognize, and the diagnosis is often made during a routine eye examination prior to the patient actually experiencing symptoms. Patient education follows, along with possible genetic counseling. It is difficult to forecast in advance how severely retinitis pigmentosa may affect one's vision in the future. I have seen cases that eventually led to blindness, but I have also followed stable adult patients who maintained good vision for years, even though they were told in childhood that they could expect to be blind by now.

However, don't automatically assume that if you are experiencing night vision problems that you have retinitis pigmentosa. Though that is a possibility, night vision problems normally have less severe underlying causes.

COMPUTER VISION SYNDROME

In a recent American Eye-Q Survey from the American Optometric Association, 46 percent of respondents reported that they spend five hours or more a day using portable electronic devices.[6] Even today's cell phones are computers that do much more than just place calls. America is certainly a "connected" society and a significant part of our social lives and work involves computers. It is no surprise, then, that computers can have negative effects on our eyes. Fortunately, many computer-related eye problems can be resolved with the proper tools and education.

Computer vision syndrome (CVS) is a combination of symptoms caused by computer use, including headaches, eye strain, and dry eyes. A national survey of optometrists by the *Journal of the American Optometric Association* discovered that 14 percent of patients complain of eye or vision-related symptoms as a result

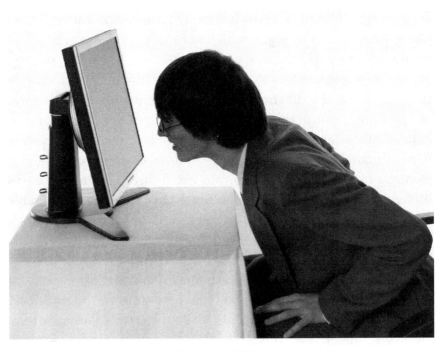

Computer Vision

of computer use.[7] Computers often require us to sit in the same position for great lengths of time, staring at a self-illuminated screen, and often at very tiny print or spreadsheets. Just like muscle fatigue and tiredness result from working our bodies all day, the eye muscles tire and become fatigued in the same way. Headaches (particularly in the forehead area) are a regular symptom that may indicate your eyes are working too hard. As the internal eye muscles fatigue, they can't hold the focus as well. Lifting a one-pound weight is not much of a challenge for most people, but carrying that same weight around all day fatigues most everyone. The same follows for the eyes. Focusing images from a computer on the retina causes the ciliary muscles to flex and contract. They are adept at this, but not for sustained periods of time, and they tire just as our other muscles do.

The Rule of 20-20-20

For every twenty minutes of computer use, take a twenty-second break, and focus the eyes on something twenty feet away. This is like putting that one-pound weight down for a moment, shaking the muscle out, and then resuming use. It gives the eyes a brief rest that prolongs the time before they become tired. Following this rule will go a long way to alleviating eye strain at the computer.

Burning, Tearing, and Dry Eyes

Dry eyes while using the computer (particularly in contact lens wearers) is a significant problem that millions of people suffer from each day. The reason for this symptom is pretty simple. The front surface of our eyes requires a healthy layer of tears to maintain proper focus, lubrication, oxygen, and nourishment. The tears are essential to proper focusing, and without them images on the computer become blurry. Each time we blink, the eyelid distributes a fresh layer of tears over the eyes. We normally blink twenty times a minute, which is about every three seconds. When working on a computer or concentrating, however, our blink rate drops to only about a third that amount (one blink every ten seconds). The prolonged exposure of the front of the eye to air allows for tear evaporation between blinks. Subsequently, it becomes uncomfortable to blink because of the reduced lubrication between the eye and eyelid.

One answer is to consciously remember to blink on a regular basis. Artificial tears are also widely available over the counter and are great to keep on hand near the computer, particularly when you wear contact lenses. I advise patients to use artificial tears every few hours during the day while at the computer, even before symptoms begin. Keeping the eyes moist will prolong the time before experiencing dry eye symptoms or possibly prevent them altogether.

The hallmark symptom of dry eyes is a burning sensation. Often, the dryness causes a gritty or sandy feeling despite not actually having anything in the eyes. Another seemingly unusual symptom is excessive tearing. Tearing seems to be the opposite of dry eyes. However, when the eyes are so dry that they feel gritty and burn, the brain receives a signal from the ocular nerves that there is something foreign in the eyes. The brain responds by signaling to "turn on the tears" to wash out any foreign bodies.

If you experience dry eyes away from the computer, other organic issues with a larger underlying cause may be at fault. An eye doctor can help diagnose the problem and effectively treat it (see Chapter 7 for more information).

Computer Glare

Glare is often an unidentified source of discomfort and eye strain at the computer. Keep the computer images being viewed at the highest contrast possible. When feasible, the most desirable contrast setting is black text on a white background. In addition, adjust the monitor's illumination to match that of the environment. Try to avoid having the monitor dimmer or brighter than the overall ambient light. Glare is not caused by the light emanating from your computer as much as it is from light external to your monitor being reflected in the monitor's surface. For options on reducing computer glare, see the section earlier in this chapter on glare.

Lastly, consider a thorough computer-related vision examination. A competent eye doctor will proactively ask about each person's computer usage and habits. However, even if not specifically asked, tell your doctor about your computer usage habits and ask what can be done to help. Today, there are millions of people benefitting from eyeglasses specifically designed for computer usage. Bifocal or progressive lens wearers who use a computer more than two hours a day may benefit from a separate pair of computer glasses designed specifically for that task. Computer eyeglasses make tangible improvements toward ocular comfort and work efficiency.

PART THREE

YOUR AGING EYES

CHAPTER 6
CHILDREN'S EYE ISSUES

The majority of children are born with normal and healthy eyes, but when problems do exist, non-verbal infants are obviously unable to communicate their complaints and symptoms to others. Toddlers and children who *are* verbal may accept a symptom as "normal" because they are unaware of what is considered abnormal. A visual or ocular health problem diagnosis often comes from an astute parent who suspects a problem may exist or, when a problem is less obvious, a pediatrician or eye care provider may first discover it.

Many ocular dysfunctions have no obvious symptoms and cannot be diagnosed without proper instrumentation. Without early intervention, many conditions such as amblyopia may irreversibly affect the child for the remainder of his or her life. However, early diagnosis and treatment may rectify many problems early on. The American Optometric Association recommends that all infants have their first eye examination by six months of age.[8] Fortunately, pediatricians screen for vision and ocular health problems at routine check-ups and will refer the infant to an eye care specialist as needed. All children, regardless of risk or symptoms, should have a comprehensive vision and ocular health examination by an eye care provider before beginning first grade, or by age five.

EXCESSIVE TEARING

The nasolacrimal duct is the "drain pipe" in each of our four eye-lids that allows the proper transportation of tears away from our eyes into our nasal passages. Our noses "run" when we cry because tears drain into the nose through the eyelids as well as running down the face.

After we're born, our eyes don't begin producing tears for at least a couple of weeks, and it may also take several weeks for the nasolacrimal canal (which contains the duct) to fully open. Dacryostenosis is a condition affecting up to 30 percent of infants in which the nasolacrimal duct does not fully open, preventing proper tear drainage. The main symptom of this blockage is excessive tearing, since the tears overflow out of the eye rather than draining properly into the nasal passages. Often, there is discharge and crusting around the eyes when the nasolacrimal canal is blocked. Discharge from the eye may be mistakenly diagnosed as an eye infection because the symptoms are alike. If dacryostenosis is misdiagnosed as an eye infection, repeated treatments for the same "eye infection" without improvement alerts the doctor to consider the alternate diagnosis of dacryostenosis.

Though not always, dacryostenosis can lead to an infection of the eyelid itself. This internal eyelid infection is called dacryocystitis, and it presents as a swollen, red, tender, and painful area around the nose and affected eyelid. Dacryocystitis is treated with oral antibiotics by the child's pediatrician or a pediatric eye-care provider.

If the drainage is blocked but not infected, it still needs to be opened so that tears may drain properly. After the diagnosis of dacryostenosis, the initial treatment is to gently massage the affected area on the side of the nose and eyelid three times a day. Over the course of several days, the massages will often successfully break up the internal blockage and allow tears to begin normal flow through the canal. It's also helpful to use a clean, warm washcloth to wipe away any discharge that may dry and accumulate around the eyelids. Keeping this area clean and free of debris can help to prevent dacryocystitis from developing or returning.

If nasolacrimal massages prove unsuccessful at opening the blockage, the doctor will probe the canal and attempt to break open or flush out the blockage. Depending on the age of the child, this probing can be done while the child is awake with local anesthesia in the form of eyedrops or the child may require general anesthesia. If all other attempts at restoring the communication between the eyelid and nasal passages are unsuccessful, eyelid surgery may be required by an oculoplastic surgeon.

While it is uncommon, excessive tearing and eyelid pain may be caused by infantile glaucoma, not dacryostenosis or dacryocystitis. It is difficult to properly diagnose these conditions, so it is important that a health-care provider examine a child who is exhibiting these symptoms.

CONJUNCTIVITIS

The conjunctiva is a clear, thin mucous membrane that covers the whites of the eyes and the underside of the eyelids. This tissue is susceptible to infection by bacteria and viruses just as our sinuses, ears, and throats may be infected. Commonly referred to as "pinkeye," conjunctivitis comes in many forms and from many causes. The most common causes of conjunctivitis in children are bacteria, viruses, or allergies. Eye irritants such as pool chlorine, smoke, shampoo, and soaps may also cause conjunctivitis.

Newborns may develop bacterial conjunctivitis as they pass through the birth canal if the mother has gonorrhea or chlamydia. These sexually transmitted diseases are bacterial in nature and often the mother is treated during pregnancy prior to giving birth, preventing transmission to the newborn. However, the mother's sexually transmitted disease diagnosis is not always made prior to giving birth. For this reason, antibiotic ointment is administered to infants' eyes just after birth to prophylactically treat any bacteria that may have passed to the newborn.

In all types of conjunctivitis, the eyes are uncomfortable and the whites of the eyes are red, giving anywhere from a light pink up to a bright red appearance (hence, the name "pink-eye"). Symptoms of conjunctivitis may include frequent tearing, pain, light sensitivity, discharge, swelling and/or matting shut of the eyelids, and itching.

The most common type of conjunctivitis in children is caused by bacteria. The bacteria that cause eye infections are often the same ones that cause sinus and ear infections. Infections involving these different organ systems may all occur simultaneously.

Bacterial Conjunctivitis

Bacterial conjunctivitis can develop quickly and may cause significant crusting of the eyelids, yellow to green discharge of pus during the day, and matting of the eyelids so that they are difficult to open upon waking in the morning. Bacterial conjunctivitis is contagious and is easily spread to the unaffected eye and to other people. I advise patients with bacterial (and viral) conjunctivitis to behave the same way they would when they have a cold: wash your hands frequently, don't shake hands with others, and don't share towels, washcloths, and pillowcases with others. Also, don't rub or wipe the infected eye and then rub the unaffected eye, as it will become cross-infected.

Parents should consider keeping children home from school for forty-eight hours after starting antibiotic eyedrops to prevent the infection from spreading to other people. Conjunctivitis spreads quickly through schools and daycare centers, but the spread of pink-eye is mitigated if the child stays home for a couple of days.

Bacterial conjunctivitis will likely go away on its own within two weeks, but treatment with prescription antibiotic eyedrops clears the infection in half the time or less and reduces the exposure of others to the contagious infection. Visiting your child's eye-care provider or pediatrician at the first sign of an eye infection is strongly recommended.

Viral Conjunctivitis

Viral conjunctivitis has many of the same symptoms as bacterial conjunctivitis, but whereas viral eye infections make the eyes look pink in color, bacterial infections make the eyes more red than pink. Another difference between viral and bacterial infections is that viral infections cause more excessive tearing, with little to no pus. Bacterial infections usually involve heavy amounts of pus.

Viral eye infections may last anywhere from a few days up to several months. Like all viruses, there are not many treatment options for this type of infection other than cold compresses to soothe the eyes. Infrequently, a doctor may use steroid eye drops in an attempt to make a very uncomfortable patient feel better, but it does not alter the course of the virus. A newer treatment option that is "off-label"—not specifically approved by the U.S. Food and Drug Administration (FDA)—and has reportedly excellent results is a diluted solution of Betadine, which is directly applied to the eye as an eyedrop in the doctor's office. Betadine is an iodine solution that is widely used as a sterilization preparation on the skin prior to a surgical procedure.

Allergic Conjunctivitis

Allergic conjunctivitis is more common in adults than children, but it may occur at any age. Allergic conjunctivitis occurs in a rapid fashion as the result of exposure to pollen, grass, dust mites, chemicals, certain foods, or any other substance to which you are allergic. It can be either acute or chronic.

Acute allergic conjunctivitis is the eye's rapid (and exaggerated) response to an allergen. The hallmark symptoms are itchiness of the eyes, redness, and sometimes swelling of the eyelids. If the itchiness worsens when you rub your eyes, it is likely an allergic reaction. Depending on the severity, the eyelids may swell due to the excessive inflammatory response enough to cause them to shut. Acute allergic reactions may involve other areas of the body in addition to the eyes, so it's wise to seek medical attention. Once the diagnosis of allergic conjunctivitis is made, oral antihistamines such as Benadryl (though this causes drowsiness), Claritin, Dimetapp, or Chlor-Trimeton get at it from the inside. Cold compresses directly on the affected eye(s) will help, too. Wrap a few ice cubes in a washcloth and hold it on the closed eye for intervals of five to ten minutes, as often as possible until the swelling subsides. Severe allergic reactions may require prescription medications or epinephrine injections prescribed by your health-care provider.

Chronic allergic conjunctivitis is typically a less severe but longer lasting manifestation of the same signs and symptoms. Acute conjunctivitis normally occurs when there's a limited exposure to the offending agent and then it's removed, whereas chronic conjunctivitis is a result of prolonged exposure to the allergen. Chronic allergic conjunctivitis frequently occurs when someone lives with a pet they are allergic to or due to the seasonal hayfever that occurs in the Spring and Fall months in many areas of the country. Over-the-counter anti-allergy medications are a good way to begin treating chronic allergies. However, prescription tablets, liquid, nasal spray, and eyedrop medications are very effective in the management of chronic allergies.

STRABISMUS (CROSSED EYES OR LAZY EYE)

There are six eye muscles attached to each eyeball inside the skeletal orbit that guide the movements of our eyes in all directions. The muscles of each eye are controlled by three nerves: the oculomotor, trochlear, and abducens. As in our arms and legs, the eye muscles have actions that oppose each other—muscles for looking left and opposing muscles for looking right. Opposing muscles keep the corresponding muscle group in check. Unless all eye muscles are properly balanced, it is difficult for the two eyes to line up properly. One faulty nerve or muscle upsets the entire balance of eye alignment and binocularity.

Normal alignment of the eyes is referred to as orthotropia. Strabismus occurs when the two eyes act independently of one

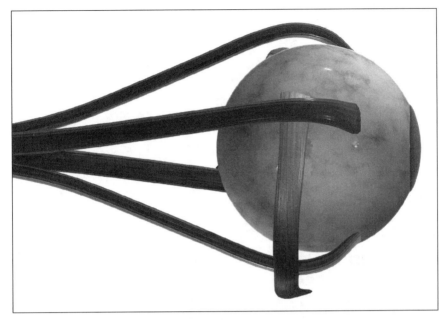

Extraocular Muscles

another and don't align. It may be present intermittently or constantly. Occasional "crossed-eyes" and constant "crossed-eyes" have differing visual ramifications and solutions. There are three terms used to define the direction of misaligned eyes in strabismus:

- Exotropia—An outward-turning eye that causes a horizontal misalignment of the eyes away from the nose (occasional or permanent).

- Esotropia—An inward-turning eye that causes a horizontal misalignment of the eyes toward the nose (occasional or permanent).

- Hypertropia—One eye higher than the other, causing a vertical misalignment of the eyes (occasional or permanent).

Strabismus may also have both vertical and horizontal components at the same time, resulting in a diagonal misalignment of the eyes.

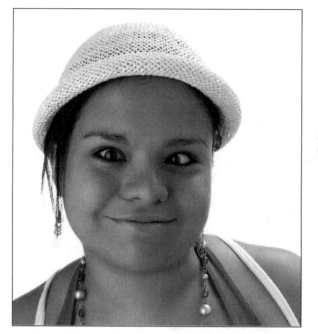

Strabismic
Esotropia

Exotropia, esotropia, and hypertropia are further defined as constant or intermittent. And, constant or intermittent crossed-eyes are also defined by being limited to one eye or alternating. When strabismus is said to be alternating, the misalignment may switch between eyes so that they alternate which eye points in the wrong direction. To further complicate matters, all types of strabismus may manifest only when looking at one focal distance and not others. For example, focal distance–related types of strabismus (such as convergence insufficiency, which we'll explore a little later) only manifest when working on a computer or reading but not while looking at a distance.

Under normal binocular vision, two images travel toward the brain, one from each eye. The brain then "fuses" the separate images received from the right and left eyes and combines them into a single image and creates depth perception. Covering one eye still allows vision of course, but the brain is receiving only half of its normal visual input, and only very limited information about depth perception is then available. In strabismus, the brain handles the images from the right and left eye differently than in normal binocular vision.

When strabismus causes the two images from the eyes to be so different that the brain can't fuse them into one image, one of two possible outcomes occurs. The first result is double vision, seeing two separate images at the same time. Certainly, this is not a desirable situation. The brain is developed enough to know that double vision is bad, so in many cases the second result, image suppression, will occur instead of double vision. In suppression, the brain can selectively ignore the image from one eye and disregard it so that double vision is averted. Usually, suppression is a benefit, but sometimes it may stunt development of the eyes in the young. If suppression occurs on a regular basis, it may result in a visually underdeveloped eye, or amblyopia.

In the first six months of life, it is developmentally normal to observe intermittent eye turns in all infants. If the eye turn is constant before six months of age, or intermittent after six months, a visit to a pediatric eye care provider is warranted for further evaluation. Do not delay this evaluation, as undiagnosed eye turns may irreversibly block eyesight development in children.

Types of Strabismus

Infantile Esotropia

Infantile esotropia is a constant misalignment of the eyes whereby an eye turns toward the nose. This type of esotropia is frequently hereditary in nature and can be very pronounced. The same eye may constantly turn in or the misaligned eye may alternate between the left and the right. Infantile esotropia will typically be noticeable before six months of age, and it usually requires surgery to correct. Multiple eye muscle surgeries over several years may be required to adjust the eye alignment as the child grows. Strabismus surgery makes a cosmetic improvement to the eye turn, but having surgery may also help the visual system fully develop properly and increase the chances that the affected eye can reach full eyesight potential.

Alternating esotropia is less harmful to the development of the child's future eyesight since the eyes take turns seeing clearly, and neither eye is "suppressed" for lengthy periods of time. On the other hand, esotropia constantly affecting one eye generates image suppression indefinitely. Constant vision suppression in the same eye adversely affects visual development. Averting this developmental problem is not dependent on having surgery. Patching or "blurring" the good eye (with prescription eyedrops) is an effective way to force the suppressed eye to come back "online" and start working. Once infantile esotropia is diagnosed, the eye-care provider will likely prescribe eye-patching therapy or dilating eyedrop use. By forcing the normally suppressed eye to work several hours a day, normal vision development has the opportunity to still occur in both eyes. Temporarily patching the good eye in an attempt to help the bad one does not harm the good eye, provided that the patching is not constant.

Accommodative Esotropia

When reading or viewing an object up close, the eyes naturally turn in slightly, in a process called convergence. Viewing near objects also requires the internal eye muscles (the ciliary muscles) to flex and focus the internal physiological lens in a process called accommodation. Eye convergence and accommodation are two processes that are tied to one another neurologically. As one process occurs, the other occurs simultaneously.

An eye that is farsighted has the ability to "dial in" some prescription compensation. This is the body's attempt to naturally balance out farsightedness on its own, though that is not the normal physiology of how the eye should work. Since the process of accommodation occurs even at times it really shouldn't, the convergence process that is tied to accommodation also kicks in, causing the eyes to turn in toward each other, and the result is accommodative esotropia.

Accommodative esotropia rarely requires surgery. The good news is that once the underlying farsightedness responsible for the esotropia is addressed by eyeglasses or contact lenses, the accommodative system returns to normal, and the convergence (esotropia) goes away. The parents are happy because the esotropia disappears while the glasses are on, and the child is happy because their vision is clearer and more comfortable. The newly prescribed glasses may be single vision or bifocal lenses, depending on the individual's needs.

Convergence Insufficiency

Convergence insufficiency is among the most common types of eye muscle dysfunctions. Diagnosis and treatment of convergence insufficiency can often make significant improvements to one's quality of life. Reports vary widely, but the prevalence of convergence insufficiency has been reported at up to 13 percent of the pediatric population in the United States. Under normal circumstances, the eyes converge while reading or performing near work; in convergence insufficiency, the eyes don't turn inward as they should. The eye muscles fight and strain to turn the eyes inward but are inadequate.

Symptoms of convergence insufficiency include:

- Eyestrain (especially when reading)

- Headaches

- Blurred vision or double vision

- Poor concentration and trouble remembering what was read

- Squinting, rubbing, closing, or covering one eye

- Sleepiness while reading

- Short attention span

- Words move, jump, swim, or float on the page

- Problems with motion sickness

A skilled eye-care provider usually suspects convergence insufficiency based solely on the history and complaints of the patient and parent. Exam room testing will confirm the diagnosis, and an action plan will be prescribed, depending on the severity of the insufficiency. The fastest way to relieve the symptoms of this condition is a pair of eyeglasses designed for near vision use only.

Reading glasses for convergence insufficiency incorporate prisms ground into the lenses. These prisms act to bend light outward to the eyes that are not properly turning in. Rather than the eyes being forced to struggle, the prisms bend light outward to arrive where the eyes already are, without requiring convergence. This takes the demand off the eye muscles and allows clear, binocular vision without the previous struggle. Reading glasses with prisms will normally resolve the symptoms very quickly. Be aware, though, that the eyes usually don't require the prism at distance, so the reading glasses can actually make the distance vision uncomfortable. For this reason, the person with convergence insufficiency almost always removes the glasses to see far away.

Various forms of vision therapy are also often effective ways of treating convergence insufficiency. Some people's eyes respond well to training of the eye muscles in order to strengthen their ability to converge. The most common method of vision therapy is called "Pencil Push-Ups." Pencil Push-Up Therapy (PPT) has been shown to have high success rates in reducing the symptoms of convergence insufficiency, but it requires perseverance on the part of both the parents and child to be effective. Remembering and sticking to the training regimen becomes tedious quickly, especially for a child.

PPT consists simply of holding a pencil with the eraser side up at arm's length from the eyes. The patient slowly brings the eraser in a straight line toward their nose while maintaining focus on the eraser as long as possible. This exercise is performed for 10–20 minutes a day, twice a day, for several weeks. In many cases, the patient is able to gradually bring the pencil eraser closer to their nose before the image blurs and convergence ceases. Strengthening the eye muscles in this way is an adjunct, and sometimes eventually a replacement, for the prism reading glasses.

Hypertropia

Hypertropia is a misalignment of the eyes vertically. Like other misalignments of the eyes, hypertropia may alternate eyes or remain constant in the same eye. Hypertropias are often subtle, and do not require intervention if there aren't any symptoms such as double vision.

Eyeglasses with prisms can help a mildly hypertropic patient maintain binocular vision. Unfortunately, vertical deviations of the eyes do not respond to vision therapy and the eyes can't be "trained" to come back into alignment. If prism glasses insufficiently correct either the functional or cosmetic concerns of a vertical eye turn, then eye muscle surgery is usually warranted. Individuals with a mild vertical deviation of the eyes may acquire a constant head tilt toward the side of the higher eye, although they may not even be aware they are tilting their head. This is a way for the eyes to realign horizontally to avoid eye muscle strain and double vision. Eye care providers are trained to detect this sometimes subtle compensation and know to test for associated problems.

Paralytic Strabismus

Most of the previously discussed types of strabismus occur because of some type of hereditary or congenital dysfunction of the eyes. However, strabismus may be acquired later in life, after normal eye muscle function has been present. Paralytic strabismus occurs because of some interruption of normal eye movement, usually neurological or muscular in nature. In some cases, such as thyroid disease or a tumor in the orbit, an obstruction in the orbit itself prevents the eye from moving properly, even though the nerve signal and muscles are normal. Only an evaluation by a health-care provider, and sometimes tests such as a CAT scan, can accurately diagnose the source of the problem.

Paralytic strabismus is sometimes temporary, as in the case of diabetes. Diabetics may temporarily lose function of an eye muscle that may last for several months and then spontaneously resolve. No permanent ocular damage occurs as a result, though double vision is disconcerting to say the least. There are many effective ways to deal with this temporary double vision. In other cases, a spontaneous onset of an eye turn may indicate a more serious problem such as a tumor or stroke, an aneurysm, or a degenerative disease such as multiple sclerosis. Though your situation may not be the "worst case scenario," do not delay in having a newly acquired eye turn medically evaluated.

Severe trauma to the head or face may damage one or more of the eye muscles or nerves, which may result in an eye muscle imbalance. Traumatically induced eye turns sometimes only manifest in certain gaze positions but not all. The fourth cranial nerve (the troclear nerve) controls the superior oblique muscle in each eye and is particularly susceptible to damage in severe head trauma. If a fourth nerve palsy is diagnosed subsequent to trauma, it is normally observed for six months or more prior to the decision to intervene surgically, as many of these imbalances resolve on their own over time.

AMBLYOPIA

Unlike most other parts of the body, the visual system is only partially developed at birth. As vision occurs in each eye, the visual system and associated neurological components continue to develop and form during the first six months of life. If a developing eye is not exposed to clear images during those first six months, the neurological pathways between the eye and the brain stop developing before they reach their full potential. *Amblyopia* is the term used when vision is partially or fully obscured because of a communication problem between the eye and the brain. The severity of amblyopia varies greatly from one person to the next: it may mean that the affected eye struggles to see the 20/20 line on the eye chart clearly, or it could be much worse, such as difficulty seeing 20/400 (typically the "big E" on the eye chart). Sometimes, amblyopia may be so mild that it isn't detected until adulthood.

Reduced vision from amblyopia is not normally the result of defective ocular anatomy. An amblyopic eye typically has the same internal and external anatomic appearance as a fully functional eye. Instead, the complicated neurological system that comprises our visual system is responsible for the vision problem.

Amblyopia is attributed to three different reasons, categorized as strabismic, refractive, or deprivation.

Strabismic amblyopia is the result of an eye turn (in any direction) that was constant in the same eye, typically from birth. In an attempt to prevent double vision caused by an eye turn, the brain suppresses (turns off) the image received by the misaligned eye. Constant suppression prevents the full development of the eye, resulting in strabismic amblyopia. If diagnosed early, strabismic amblyopia may be averted or even reversed via patching therapy.

Refractive amblyopia often occurs when there is a sizeable difference in refractive error (myopia, hyperopia, and/or astigmatism) between the two eyes. One of the two eyes usually sees well, but the eye with the large refractive error does not. The image quality reaching the eye with a high, uncorrected prescription is poor, and visual development is retarded.

Deprivation amblyopia is the least common type of amblyopia. Unlike strabismic and refractive amblyopia, deprivation amblyopia affects both eyes. This may happen as the result of obscured vision from cataracts in both eyes (sometimes present at birth,) or a high refractive error in both eyes that goes undiagnosed. If the cataracts are removed in early childhood, or glasses are prescribed early enough, the visual system will resume development and long-term amblyopia may be avoided or mitigated.

Patching Therapy

With strabismic or refractive amblyopia, there is a window of time whereby patching the "good eye" forces the amblyopic eye to work. Placing an eye patch (or using some other means of vision obstruction) over the non-amblyopic eye allows the non-dominant, amblyopic eye the opportunity to work and see on its own. Ideally, if the amblyopic eye is given a visual stimulus long enough, it may eliminate or lessen permanently reduced vision. The human visual system is considered "plastic" up through age ten. Beyond that, the visual system is fairly unchangeable, and patching therapy success rates decline dramatically. It is not entirely useless for an adult amblyopic patient to attempt patching therapy, but the odds of success are low.

In a typical patching therapy regimen, the patient is instructed to wear an eye patch over the good eye for 6–10 hours a day during times of visual activity. This includes times they are performing a visually demanding task like reading, watching TV, or playing video games. It is important to have several hours a day without any patch to allow the unaffected eye to have time to be used also. Provided that it is allowed to see unobstructed for several hours a day, no harm will be done by patching the "good eye."

Children, particularly infants, are notoriously challenging to keep an eye patch on. An alternate method of obscuring or "patching" the good eye temporarily is through the use of prescription eyedrops that will cause the pupil to dilate. These drops subsequently blur the image in that eye for a specified period of time. The doctor will recommend the best option for the particular situation.

COLOR BLINDNESS (COLOR DEFICIENCY)

Blindness is not a term I like to use unless someone is truly without vision. The term *color deficiency* is a more accurate description. There is a misconception that a color-deficient person perceives vision in black and white only, similar to a black-and-white television; however, this is untrue. Instead, most individuals who are "color blind" actually have an altered sense of color among certain wavelengths only. In a rare form of color deficiency called monochromacy, vision truly is only in shades of grey. Ninety-nine

FACTORS THAT MAY AFFECT COLOR VISION

CONDITIONS/DISEASES

Cataracts	Macular degeneration
Diabetes	Retinoblastoma (in children)
Kallman's syndrome	Parkinson's disease
Leber's hereditary optic neuropathy	

MEDICATIONS

Myambutol (arthritis medication)	Oral contraceptives
Ibuprofen (Advil)	Digitalis
Naproxen (Aleve)	Chloroquine (Hydroxychloroquine)
Estradiol	Plaquenil

percent of color deficiencies mainly affect the colors red and green. These red-green affected individuals still have some color vision, similar to a normally sighted individual, but they have a difference of perception in the red and green color wavelengths. To a red-green deficient individual, red colors are perceived more closely to grey, while greens may look somewhere between white and blue. Approximately 1 percent of color deficiencies affect the blue and yellow colors.

Color deficiencies predominantly manifest in males. Reports vary, though it's believed that 5–10 percent of the male population has some color deficiency, while fewer than 1 percent of females are thought to manifest a color deficiency.[9]

Most color deficiencies are present at birth, but a color deficiency may also develop later in life. Congenital color deficiencies are genetically inherited and usually have a predictable pattern of inheritance. Though men normally express the color deficiency trait, it is inherited predominantly through the mother. Women who carry the color deficiency trait often don't manifest the deficiency themselves. Color deficiencies may be acquired later in life due to many conditions or medications.

The retina is comprised of two types of perception cells, rods and cones. The cells responsible for color vision are the cones, and there are three types: blue, green, and red. The three color cell types combine their visual inputs to allow us to see a spectrum of colors. Color deficiencies can originate from many neurological areas, but most deficiencies are the result of the cone cells' inability to properly receive and process the different wavelengths of light in the eyes.

Color vision is tested in a number of ways, including many free online screening tests. Since there are so many variable factors, color vision is best tested by an eye-care professional. The standard color vision screening method is the Ishihara Color Plate Book. If a more detailed study of color vision is required, the Farnsworth color vision test is often used.

Most people with color-deficient eyesight navigate their way through life quite well, albeit with some embarrassing moments—with mismatched clothing selections, for example. However, certain scenarios may be dangerous for color-deficient individuals, such as horizontally oriented traffic lights. The typical vertical orientation of a traffic signal allows a color-deficient individual to know that the top light is "stop," even if they can't recognize that it's red, but a horizontally oriented signal may be confusing. Professions that require proper color discernment, such as electricians (color-coded wires) and pilots (color-coded instrument panels and runway lights), obviously present a problem.

While various specialty eyeglasses and contact lenses designed to help color-deficient individuals have come and gone over the years, no single design has been considered a "runaway" success. These specialty lenses do not restore normal color vision to a color-deficient individual, but many users report that they can more easily detect different "heats" or subtle shade differences in colors. Keep in mind that specialty lenses for color deficiency are sometimes costly and experimental. I believe it is worthwhile to explore these options with your doctor, but do so with the idea of it possibly being an unsuccessful experiment.

NYSTAGMUS

Nystagmus is a family of eye conditions that consist of involuntary, often very rapid, jumpy eye movements horizontally or vertically. Rather than the eyes being able to "lock" onto a visual target, they continue to move, even when trying to gaze upon a fixed object. Individuals with nystagmus are often born with it, but it may be acquired later in life. The effects are usually limited to the cosmetic and a self-conscious sense of differently functioning eyes, but nystagmus usually has little effect on visual ability. In other cases, nystagmus may have significant visual implications or have other serious underlying causes, such as trauma or neurological dysfunction.

Acquired nystagmus may result from certain medications (particularly epilepsy drugs,) brain tumors, multiple sclerosis, trauma, or other rare conditions. If the underlying cause is modifiable, nystagmus may be treatable. There are fewer treatments available for individuals born with nystagmus, but sometimes eyeglasses or contact lenses may help.

Given the wide variety of underlying causes, classifications, and treatments of nystagmus, this condition should be evaluated by an eye doctor.

READING AND ACADEMIC PERFORMANCE— THE VISION LINK

Most classroom learning occurs through our eyesight. Our visual system is one of the largest driving factors in a successful education. It is estimated that 10 percent of school-aged children have undiagnosed visual problems and are likely suffering academically as a result. Of course, not all learning problems are related to eyesight, but many are, so analysis of the visual system is an important step in determining the source of any learning disabilities.

Conditions such as dyslexia, attention-deficit/hyperactivity disorder (ADHD), and other learning disabilities are often elusive diagnoses since each child will manifest their symptoms differently.

A thorough visual system analysis is critical to fully understanding the underlying problems. Your eye-care provider will communicate with other health-care providers, such as the child's pediatrician, psychologist, and school nurse, and combine all findings in order to better arrive at an accurate diagnosis. In many cases, the visual system does not play a role in the learning disability, but this should be determined after an examination.

Refractive conditions of the eyes, particularly farsightedness and astigmatism, can make near visual tasks very difficult for sustained periods of time. These visual conditions may allow the individual's eyesight to test well at a distance or even at near for short periods of time. A condition called "latent hyperopia" is particularly insidious to proper functioning of the visual system, since it can be

Vision Therapy

Vision therapy (VT) is loosely defined as medically directed eye exercises to improve the eyes' functioning, comfort, focusing, visual perception, and efficiency. (Vision therapy should not be confused with what's offered on TV infomercials advertising eye exercise programs that supposedly allow you to improve your eyesight enough to throw away your glasses forever.) A vision therapy program consists of an eye doctor–directed set of progressive exercises and routines tailored to improve previously diagnosed weak visual skills. VT sessions are normally scheduled once or twice a month over several months and consist of baseline testing, home eye exercises (often computer software based), and progressive testing in-office to monitor improvement. VT can often improve conditions such as convergence insufficiency, provide athletic vision enhancement, and help brain trauma patients.

According to the American Optometric Association (AOA), vision therapy can improve visual efficiency and processing, which allows a child to be more responsive to educational instruction. VT an intermittent problem. Latent hyperopia is farsightedness that is partially compensated for by the eye muscles working overtime. It is only diagnosed with the use of prescription eyedrops, which temporarily prevent the visual system from over-compensating. This problem is simply resolved with the proper eyeglass prescription, and often dramatic improvements in academic performance result. Other types of refractive errors may also be the source of the problem, and they can be diagnosed during a vision examination.

Ocular functioning, such as eye tracking and improper eye movements, may be the cause of academic problems, even if there is no need for prescription eyeglasses or contact lenses. Many children with academic problems related to vision may have 20/20 sight on screening tests at school and in the pediatrician's office

is a specialty in the field of optometry, and not all optometrists are set up to practice it. However, if your optometrist detects a condition that may respond to vision therapy, a referral will be made. A great resource for finding a vision therapy doctor and learning more about VT is the College of Optometrists in Vision Development website: www.COVD.org.

Vision therapy is sometimes dismissed as "voodoo science," particularly among ophthalmologists. There is a substantial body of scientific evidence documenting the efficacy of vision therapy when applied appropriately in responsive visual conditions. If VT is suggested by an eye-care provider, I recommend asking the doctor for the names of other patients you can contact who have been successfully treated with VT for the same condition.

While my optometry practice does not provide vision therapy, I have witnessed many cases where VT has improved patients' quality of life. I have also observed several cases where VT did not provide much or any improvement. In my experience, VT works for some but not for all who undergo these programs. Nevertheless, I believe vision therapy may be an effective means to improving visual skills, and it is a worthwhile undertaking.

and appear to have "normal" eyes. This is one further reason why a comprehensive examination by an eye doctor is important starting at six months of age.

The six eye muscles around each eye are controlled by a complex set of different nerves and neurological processes. If the eye muscles are unable to direct the eyes to the proper place, even a 20/20 eye won't function properly. Eye muscle balance and strength will be assessed as part of a comprehensive vision examination. One of the most common visual disorders that results in difficulty reading is convergence insufficiency (see under "Strabismus").

For proper binocular functioning of the visual system, the eyes should line up straight ahead when looking at any object further than six feet away. In reality, each of our eyes (in a relaxed state) has a minor tendency to point in slightly different directions. These "phorias" (tendencies of the eyes to not line up together) are compensated for pretty easily by the nervous system, but excessive phorias are more difficult or impossible for our visual system to adjust for. Phorias are rarely visible to the naked eye, but phoria testing in an eye doctor's office is quite accurate. Problematic phorias can often be managed through the use of prisms ground into eyeglass lenses or by vision therapy.

SPORTS PERFORMANCE AND SAFETY

Just as in the process of learning, the ability to perform athletically is largely governed by our visual abilities. The majority of the information that we receive and process while participating in sports comes from eyesight. Beyond our normal visual acuity on the eye chart, exceptional athletes also display exceptional dynamic visual acuity:

• Depth perception

• Peripheral vision

• Eye-hand coordination and reaction time

- Visual tracking

- Selective concentration

Depth perception—Depth perception is critical in judging distances, terrain, and multiple objects relative to one another. In football, a quarterback needs excellent depth perception to make the pass at the proper distance; a baseball batter needs to dynamically judge the distance of an oncoming pitch from the mound; and a skier needs to judge the distance and depth of oncoming moguls. Depth perception is used in all sports. The simultaneous use of visual input from each eye and assimilated by the brain (binocularity) is the basis for our depth perception. If one of the eyes is obscured or not being used, fine depth perception is lost and athletic performance will almost surely suffer.

Individuals with strabismus or amblyopia who are limited to monocular vision sometimes find sports to be frustrating, and at times even embarrassing. These individuals will unfortunately find that successfully catching a pop-fly ball or making a square racquet hit on a tennis ball is a substantial challenge. Furthermore, certain sports can be troublesome even for those who have intermittent or average depth perception. In some cases of "average" depth perception, sports vision exercises and training may prove helpful in improving visual abilities.

Peripheral vision—Peripheral vision is the ability to receive and process information surrounding the visual target. Fixed and moving objects around us are constantly being registered by our peripheral vision. A race car driver needs to be able to see and process other cars (and their distances) as they move through traffic. Basketball players need to be able to see other players to their sides and rear, and identify whether they are teammates or opponents, in order to pass the ball or help on defense. When vision-correcting lenses are needed, contact lenses provide better-quality peripheral vision compared to eyeglasses, even for pickup games in the neighborhood street. Eyeglasses limit our peripheral vision to the edge of the eyeglass frame and lenses, whereas contact lenses move with the eye and provide clear optics for more than 180 degrees of vision. In fact, normal binocular vision allows up to 210 degrees of vision.

Eye-hand coordination and reaction time—Eye-hand coordination and reaction time are measures of how quickly we experience a muscular response from our visual input. The faster and more accurately we swing a hockey stick at an approaching puck, the better we can control where the puck will go. Golfing requires eye-hand coordination in order to swing the club at the proper velocity and angle to strike the ball at exactly the desired spot. The faster the neurological response the brain sends to our muscles, the more adept we are at performing a given athletic task. Reaction times and eye-hand coordination are modifiable traits that often respond well to sports vision training, and many professional athletes receive this type of training.

Visual tracking—Visual tracking is the ability to stay mentally focused on a particular target. A great example of using visual tracking is the "ball under a cup" mix-up trick. Placing a ball under one of three cups and then scrambling the cups around quickly challenges us to visually keep track of which cup the ball is under, despite all of the confusing and deceptive moves. Once you've lost track of the cup with the ball, it is virtually impossible to pick it up again. There is no "second chance" in a task like this, and the same can be true in athletic events. Visually tracking a golf ball in the sky after a drive allows you to see where the ball eventually lands. However, if you lose visual track of the ball, it's more challenging to find it again.

Selective concentration—Selective concentration is the ability to quickly receive and process incoming information and categorize it as useful or useless. The objective is to focus all of the brain's processing power and the body's actions to accomplish your goal and to "deselect" impertinent information that is being received. An example of using selective concentration is a batter not allowing the "chatter" of the crowd to distract him from the pitch. Another example is a football player directing all of his attention to receiving a ball passed to him without being distracted by the crowd, lights, and other players moving around him.

Many of these dynamic visual acuity traits can be improved with training. The American Optometric Association has a sub-chapter of optometrists called the Sports Vision Section. These sports vision optometrists are trained and educated in how to measure and teach improvement techniques to athletes. Ask your eye doctor for a recommendation or visit the AOA website: www.aoa.org/prebuilt/DrLocator/search.asp.

Vision-Correcting Options for Sports

Soft or rigid gas permeable (RGP) contact lenses are an excellent way of addressing refractive errors of the eyes. While eyeglasses afford a small amount of eye protection compared to contact lenses, the glasses can break and cause more injuries unless the eyewear is safety approved for sports. Generally, soft contact lenses are preferred over rigid gas permeable lenses because the soft lenses are more forgiving in terms of comfort and stability on the eye during sports. While great for non-sporting activities, RGPs are more readily displaced off the center of the eye in contact sports and certain environments (dry or windy weather). They are also more uncomfortable when dust or debris gets into the eye. Soft lenses are not affected nearly as much by these external factors.

The biggest advantage contact lenses provide is unobstructed peripheral vision compared to eyeglasses. Furthermore, contact lenses are not susceptible to fogging, sweat, or raindrops the same way eyeglass lenses are. In prescriptions stronger than –4.00 and +4.00 diopters, the optical clarity through contact lenses is usually superior to eyeglasses. Since the contact lens stays placed centrally over the pupil during eye movements, the center of the eye is always looking through the "optical center" of the contact lens, providing the truest and clearest prescription. Looking through the peripheral areas of an eyeglass lens in higher prescriptions induces optical aberrations, and clarity is diminished because the center of the eyeglass lens is not always directly over the center of the eye.

I am often asked by parents if their Little League or soccer-playing children are too young for contact lenses. There is no exact age that a child becomes "contact lens eligible," nor is any age too young in my opinion. Eye doctors routinely fit children of all ages in contact lenses. A child's candidacy for contact lenses is largely a function of their own desire (*not* their parents' desire), their level of responsibility, and their ability to tolerate things in close proximity to their eyes, such as a finger inserting a contact lens. It is desirable to fit a young athlete in contact lenses as early as they are able to tolerate them, since contact lenses hold so many advantages over eyeglasses in sports vision. Bear in mind that the intangible advantage of increased confidence provided by contact lenses factors into sports performance as well. Today, with the availability of single use, daily disposable contact lenses, children find it even easier to use contact lenses.

Ortho-Keratology—the gentle, short-term reshaping of the cornea by a customized RGP contact lens—is an effective way to manage certain amounts of nearsightedness and astigmatism in athletes of all ages. Even the best soft contact lenses can become dislodged in the eye, and are susceptible to dry, windy, and dusty environments. Ortho-K allows the athlete to wear the lenses overnight and to enjoy clear vision without any contact lenses or eyeglasses during the day and while participating in sports. This is particularly nice for swimmers, as wearing contact lenses in the pool is undesirable. (See more on Ortho-Keratology in Chapter 3.)

Sports and Eye Safety

Regardless of whether or not an athlete has a refractive error, measures need to be taken to protect the eyes while participating in sports. According to the AOA, sports-related eye injuries are the number one cause of eye injuries in those aged sixteen years and younger. It is estimated that 90 percent of these injuries are preventable with the proper eyewear.[10] Estimates by Prevent Blindness America place the number of sports-related eye injuries at 40,000 per year, with about one-third of those visits being children.[11]

The sports most frequently responsible for eye injuries are baseball, basketball, and racquet sports. One of the most dangerous sports to the eye is racquetball. The bony orbit around the eye typically limits a ball that hits the eye from compressing the orbit very far. However, the small diameter of a racquetball allows it to fit into the eye socket without being blocked by the bones around it, and excessive compression of the eye occurs. An eye injury from a racquetball may result in permanently losing the eye. Fingers, elbows, and collisions are sources of serious eye injuries during other sports.

Protective eyewear designed for sports usage is inexpensive insurance against permanently damaging an eye. While normal eyeglasses may provide some protection, most frames and lenses are not sturdy enough to withstand the severity of impacts that occur in sports. Safety goggles are ideal, as they are designed to minimize any visual disturbances while using them. They are made with materials that can withstand impacts and have lenses grooved so that they can only pop outward, away from the eyes. Many quality sports goggles also have side vents or anti-fog lenses so that they don't cause problems when sweating. For sports already requiring a helmet, a face shield should be used with the helmet to protect the eyes.

Sustaining an eye injury puts one at greater risk for developing a traumatic cataract. Direct trauma to the eye significantly increases the chances of developing a sight-reducing cataract months or years after the injury occurred, regardless of age. Though cataracts can usually be surgically treated, if the trauma was severe enough to cause a cataract, most likely other permanent damage has occurred as well. (For more information on traumatic eye injuries, see Chapter 9.)

Eye care providers have access to high-quality safety eyewear designed for use during sports. One brand that is commonly found is Rec Specs. Make sure that your safety eyewear meets the American Society for Testing and Materials (ASTM) standard for your sport.

CHAPTER 7

ADULT
EYE ISSUES

Our eyes perform the highly important task of providing eyesight at our beck and call. We rely on our eyes to be ready to work literally in the "blink of an eye" each morning when we wake up. However, very mild to more serious issues may occur with our eyes. From the minor nuisance of an eyelid twitch to the more life-altering dysfunction of glaucoma, awareness and preventative maintenance are the best ways we can repay our eyes for all that they provide us.

DRY EYES

Dry eye syndrome is a collection of dysfunctions related to the eye's tear system. Dry eye sounds like a simple, self-explanatory problem, but it is actually quite complex. The symptoms and treatments of dry eye syndrome vary widely. A healthy tear layer provides several vital functions to our eyes, including lubrication (to soothe the friction caused by the eyelid when we blink), optimized optics, protection, and nourishment of the eye. There are three types of tears our eyes produce: basal tears, reflex tears, and emotional tears.

- Basal tears are the normal level of wetness that our eyes should have at all times. Basal tears provide lubrication between the cornea and the eyelid, and they also act to provide protection from dust, mild fumes, bacteria, viruses, and other foreign particles.

- Exposure to strong fumes, wind, or even spicy foods causes a more robust tear response called reflex tearing. Reflex tearing works by sending out an acute burst of tears in hopes that the additional tear volume will wash away the offending foreign substances or fumes.

- Emotional tears are the flood of tears in response to mourning, weeping, or "tears of joy" that run over the eyelids onto our face and into our nasal passages.

Dry eye syndrome is primarily a dysfunction of the basal tears, as most dry eye sufferers still have normal reflex and emotional tearing. Men and women of all ages can be affected by dry eyes, and it may be acute or chronic in nature. For some, dry eye syndrome is just a minor nuisance that requires nothing more than instilling an artificial tear drop occasionally to provide relief. However, severe dry eye syndrome may be so visually disabling that the individual is functionally incapacitated and cannot carry on a normal lifestyle. Symptoms caused by dry eyes are among the most common reasons for visits to eye doctors. Fortunately, the medical community has gained a very thorough, though still evolving, understanding of this prevalent condition. In fact, there are many specialized "dry eye clinics" across the United States, predominantly found in environmentally dry areas such as Colorado and the Southwest.

Symptoms of Dry Eyes

The list of dry eye symptoms is lengthy, but several stand out as "hallmark" symptoms. These include burning of the eyes, grittiness or a "sand in the eye" feeling, and excessive tearing. The primary symptoms of dry eyes include the following:

- Intolerance to contact lens wear

- Burning

- Gritty, sandy feeling of the eyes

- Excessive tearing

- Redness of the eyes

- Blurry or fluctuating vision

- Foreign body sensation of the eyes

- Light sensitivity

- Pain in the eyes

As contrary as it sounds, excessive tearing is often a major symptom of dry eyes, caused by the irritation our eyes suffer when we blink with an inadequate tear layer. The tear layer normally cushions and lubricates the cornea from the friction of the eyelids moving across it. When the tear layer is compromised, the lack of lubrication causes the eyelid to scratch and irritate the front of the eye with each blink. Since we blink approximately twenty times a minute, it is easy to understand how quickly the eyes may become irritated.

Causes of Dry Eyes

The causes of dry eye are nearly as numerous and varied as the symptoms themselves. Dry eye syndrome may be related to the environment, organic causes, age related, or medication induced. Short- or long-term dryness is sometimes surgically induced by LASIK laser eye surgery.

The environment is a critical factor that is often at the root of dry eyes. In higher elevations, such as the mountains, humidity levels are low and the air is dry. Lower ambient humidity causes the existing tear layer to evaporate off the eye faster than normal, generating dry eye symptoms or contact lens intolerance. This is also true in other low-humidity environments, such as in the desert or in airplanes and hospitals. Just as our lips get chapped and our skin becomes dry in certain environments, the mucous membranes of the eyes dry out, too. Any condition that increases evaporation is potentially harmful to the tear layer. Wind on the face, air conditioning vents in a car, or a blowing fan all work against the basal tear layer and speed up tear evaporation. The recycled air common in airplanes and large buildings has very low humidity and often causes dry eye symptoms in individuals who don't otherwise suffer from it.

Visually demanding tasks, such as computer work and playing video games, can significantly irritate the eyes because of dryness and evaporation. When concentrating, we only blink about a third the normal amount (normal is about twenty times a minute), and when the intervals between blinks increase, the normal basal tears evaporate. This causes the eyes to become irritated. A simple treatment when this occurs is to consciously blink more often while at the computer. Frequent blinking alleviates some of the dry eye discomfort and other symptoms, such as fluctuating vision. Making a conscious effort to blink while working on a computer has helped many people.

Organic causes of dry eye are linked to underlying systemic disease or dysfunctions of the tear-producing glands. There is a solid link between dry eyes and our body's inflammatory process—a relatively new discovery about the mechanisms of dry eye that has led to more effective treatments in the last few years. Autoimmune diseases that are inflammatory in nature, such as Sjögren's syndrome, rheumatoid arthritis, scleroderma, lupus, and Graves' disease, frequently cause dry eye. Treating the dry eye component is just one part of a multi-faceted therapeutic approach in these systemic conditions.

Age-related changes in both men and women make dry eyes a more prevalent problem as we mature (although fewer men complain of dry eyes). The body's mucous membranes produce fewer secretions over time, including tears. Up to 10 percent of post-menopausal women suffer from dry eyes—as estrogen levels decrease in menopause, the prevalence of dry eye symptoms often increases. Unfortunately, hormone replacement therapy does very little to improve dry eye symptoms in post-menopausal women, so symptoms in this population are treated the same way as in others with dry eyes.

Several over-the-counter and prescription medications are known to cause dry eye symptoms. Medications such as antihistamines and decongestants are prescribed for the primary purpose of reducing mucous membrane secretions, and so they also dry the eyes. Many birth control pills commonly cause the side effect of dry eyes. In addition, some antidepressants, ACE inhibitors, beta blockers, acne medications, sleeping pills, diuretics, and antibiotics (tetracycline and doxycycline) can cause dryness of the eyes. One of the first questions an eye doctor will ask a patient with an acute onset of dry eyes is whether any medications have been changed or new ones added recently. Teenagers who start prescription treatment for acne may suddenly find their contact lenses very dry. If medications are causing dry eyes, two approaches may be taken. In consultation with the doctors, the medication may sometimes be changed or the dosage may be altered to alleviate dry eyes without losing the desired medical effect. However, if the potential risk of changing medications outweighs the benefit of improved eye lubrication and comfort, then the eye doctor will help treat the symptoms of dry eye. Do not stop medications or alter their dosage without first consulting with the prescribing doctor.

Contact lenses play a role in dry eyes. Nearly half of contact lens wearers complain of occasional dryness that they wouldn't have had otherwise. Most soft contact lenses are approximately 50 percent water, and in order for a contact lens to maintain the proper shape and desired optics, it must be fully hydrated at all times. Contact lenses have many of the characteristics of a sponge —just as sponges need to be fully saturated to take on their natural shape, a contact lens does, too. A sponge soaks up whatever moisture it can from around it in order to maintain its own saturation and, similarly, a contact lens maintains its optimal moisture levels and optics by taking tears from the eye. Depending on the molecular composition of the lens and the environment at the time, the contact lens may sap all moisture from the eye, resulting in the typical dry eye symptoms.

If the contact lens is not the source of dryness, other causes of dry eye may still make the contact lenses uncomfortable and blurry. Without adequate tear levels throughout the period of lens wear, there is no source from which the contact lens can draw moisture as it is worn. The moisture levels of the contact lenses will eventually become inadequate for the lens to perform both optically and comfortably. As the hydration of the contact lens declines, the lens subtlely changes shape and can dramatically reduce visual clarity. Redness, blurriness, and discomfort result and the lenses will need to be removed from the eyes.

Since eye dryness is the number one reason patients discontinue contact lens use, lens and solution manufacturers have worked diligently over the years at devising new products aimed at conquering the symptoms of dry eyes. Eye doctors are knowledgeable about which contact lens brands and solutions perform best for individuals with dry eye concerns. Today, many brands of contact lenses are specifically designed to have superior qualities that counter dry eyes, including Proclear Compatibles, Ciba Night & Day, Extreme H_2O, and Acuvue Oasys.

Treatment for Dry Eyes

The level of treatment for dry eyes directly corresponds to the severity of the condition and symptoms.

Mild Dry Eyes

In mild dry eyes, education about the dry eye disease is a good starting point. Controlling the environment will also help mild dry eyes: pointing fans and vents away from the face, blinking more often, running a humidifier during the winter months (40–60 percent humidity is desirable), and drinking lots of water to keep the body hydrated are all easily modifiable factors that can improve dry eye symptoms. Speaking with your eye-care and other health-care providers about the various types of medications you are using will sometimes safely allow modifications that improve the eyes' moisture levels.

In addition, there are dozens of over-the-counter artificial tear solutions that help replace the deficient tear layers in the eyes. These drops have limitations in their symptom-reducing longevity, but they do provide short-term relief and comfort for dry eyes. From the thirty or more commercially available preparations, over-the-counter artificial tears can be divided into two large groups: those that contain preservatives and those that are preservative-free. If four or fewer administrations of the artificial tears per day sufficiently control the symptoms of dry eye, preserved artificial tears are fine to use. If the artificial tears are needed more than four times a day, then preservative-free artificial tears should be used. Preserved artificial tears are less expensive and often more convenient than preservative-free drops. The disadvantage to the preserved artificial tears is the chemical preservatives may become toxic to the eye if overused. Preservative-free artificial tears are similar in chemistry to human tears and may safely be used on a nearly unlimited basis. Unfortunately though, preservative-free drops come in small vials containing only five to six drops each in order to prevent contamination. Normally the user has to carry several of these vials with them, and they are difficult to store once the non-replaceable caps are broken off.

Most of the artificial tear solutions available are in drop form with various levels of viscosity (thickness) and a few ocular oint-ments for nighttime use are available as well. The low-viscosity drops, such as Optive and Refresh Tears, provide rapid relief to the eyes, but their beneficial effects do not last long since they are not retained in the eye more than a few minutes. Drops with slightly higher viscosity (Hypotears, BionTears, Systane) are retained in the eye longer, which provides longer-lasting relief. However, some users complain of temporarily blurred vision from the drops. The highest viscosity drops (Celluvisc) provide the longest duration of ocular retention and relief, but they can cause significant blurring.

RECOMMENDED ARTIFICIAL TEARS FOR DRY EYES

SEVERITY	PRESERVED	PRESERVATIVE-FREE
Mild dry eyes	Optive	Refresh Endura; Refresh Tears
Moderate dry eyes	Systane Ultra; Blink Tears; Hypotears	
Severe dry eyes	Soothe XP	BionTears; Celluvisc (daytime use)
		Refresh PM Ointment; Tears Naturale PM Ointment (ointments for nighttime use)

Moderate Dry Eyes

People with moderate symptoms usually require artificial tear drops more than four times a day, necessitating the use of preservative-free drops. At this moderate stage, the addition of a preservative-free ointment in the eyes just prior to bedtime may be helpful. Surprisingly, many people sleep without their eyelids being fully closed, which leaves the front of the eyes exposed to the air throughout the night, causing significant dryness and irritation the following day. Lubricating ointments significantly help those with incomplete lid closure during sleep, but the ointment can also benefit people with complete lid closure.

Moderate dry eyes often respond well to adding prescription eyedrops designed to reduce inflammation to over-the-counter artificial tears. Eye doctors treat both moderate and severe dry eye with strong prescription steroid eyedrops—often Lotemax (loteprednol etabonate ophthalmic suspension) 0.5 percent—for a couple of weeks to get inflammation under control, and then switch to a milder, long-term anti-inflammatory called Restasis, cyclosporine ophthalmic emulsion 0.05 percent.

The steroid and Restasis combination anti-inflammatory therapy has proven to be very effective treatment for inflammatory dry eye. If a significant flare-up of dry eye occurs while using Restasis, the doctor may occasionally treat the dry eye again with steroids. Not all patients benefit from the prescription drops and Restasis may take from a few weeks up to several months to reach full efficacy, so it is important to stick with the doctor's prescribed treatment. As Restasis heals the damage to the cornea caused by dry eyes, pain-receptor nerves come back "online" and temporarily cause added irritation as the physiology of the eye is restored to normal. This phenomenon usually lasts only a few days, so it is worth pressing through.

While research is still evolving, some evidence shows that omega-3 fatty acids may improve tear quality and quantity. The typical American diet does not provide all the omega-3s that the body requires. Our bodies utilize omega-3s to aid in the modulation of inflammation, and since dry eye is usually inflammatory in nature, people supplementing their diet with omega-3s often experience significant improvements in their dry eye symptoms. Omega-3 fatty acids are found naturally in dark fish, particularly in salmon and tuna, as well as cod, walnuts, and flaxseed oil. Over-the-counter omega-3 dietary supplements are widely available and easy to find in grocery stores, pharmacies, and health food stores. My own experience has been that most people with dry eye who begin omega-3 supplementation report substantial improvements in their symptoms. Do not begin taking supplements without first consulting your physician, particularly if you are on blood thinners, since omega-3s can prolong blood clotting.

Severe Dry Eyes

If the previously mild and moderate dry eye treatments are not fully effective at managing all of the symptoms, it's likely the dryness is severe. Fortunately, there are effective treatments for this as well.

One popular dry eye treatment called punctal occlusion

requires some understanding of tear physiology. Tears drain from the eyes into the nasal passages through four ducts, one in each of the eyelids near the inner corners closest to the nose. The hole in each eyelid connecting to the canal is called the punctum. Approximately 80 percent of the tears drain through the two lower eyelid ducts, and the remaining tears drain through the top ducts. This direct drainage connection from the eyes to the nasal passages explains why your nose runs when you are crying, as the nasal passages drain off excess tears from the eyes via these drainage canals.

For severe dry eyes, punctal occlusion is often used to treat the condition. This nonsurgical procedure involves "plugging" the tiny drains in the eyelids, using small, nearly invisible silicone plugs. Eye doctors perform this outpatient procedure using a microscope. It is painless and reversible at any time. The majority of people receiving punctal plugs have them inserted only into the lower lids, leaving the upper lid canals open. Gravity drains most of the tears through the lower canals, so the largest benefits are received from blocking just these ducts.

While infection or allergic reactions are possible with punctal plugs, they are extremely rare and treatable. Silicone is a benign substance that rarely generates an allergic response. The plugs may eventually come out by themselves, although it is rare for it to happen in both eyelids simultaneously. This allows patients to realize that a plug has come out, as the symptoms of dry eye suddenly increase in one eye.

Depending on the cause of the severe dry eye, oral antibiotics may be prescribed to help keep the oil glands of the eyelids functioning properly. Just as blocked oil glands in the skin cause acne, the oil glands of the eyelids may prevent the proper production of oil for the tear layer. If the oily layer of the tears is insufficient or missing entirely, the watery part of the tears will evaporate off of the eye faster than normal, leading to dry eye. In the most severe dry eyes, oral anti-inflammatory medications may be utilized to treat the symptoms. Also, special "moisture goggles" can be used during the day and while sleeping. The moisture goggles provide a seal around the edges so that a greenhouse-like effect is created around the eyes. The humidity of the air contacting the eyes can remain high because evaporating tears are unable to escape. A tightly fitting pair of sunglasses will also create some of the same effect.

A last resort in treating dry eye is a surgical procedure to tie the outer edges of the eyelids together, narrowing the distance between the upper and lower eyelids. This decreases the surface area of the front of the eye, allowing less exposed tissue to be irritated and less surface area from which the tears will evaporate.

While no "cure" exists, there are many effective ways to manage the discomfort and inconvenience of dry eyes. Don't think that you have to live with it or that it's just another condition to adjust to as you mature. Your eye-care provider is ready to help manage your dry eye condition but you must make sure to mention your concerns at your visit, as the diagnosis is often triggered by the patient's history and not what the doctor observes in the examination alone.

PREGNANCY AND THE EYES

Pregnancy affects nearly all parts of a woman's body in some way, and the eyes are no exception. Fortunately, the ocular side effects of pregnancy are rarely serious, unless they are accompanied by additional underlying conditions such as gestational diabetes or high blood pressure. Nearly all of the benign ocular changes that occur during pregnancy return to normal postpartum.

It is common and normal for a pregnant woman to experience blurriness and changes to her vision prescription throughout pregnancy. Just as swollen ankles and bloating frequently occur, the cornea may swell from excess fluid accumulation during pregnancy. The microscopically swollen cornea causes a shift in the vision prescription because the cornea is thickened by the fluid. Though it can be dramatic in some women, the vision prescription shift is usually minor. Because the prescription shift will reverse postpartum, the decision to update the eyeglass and contact lens prescriptions are made on a case-by-case basis with the eye doctor. Factors such as the amount of shift, the current week of pregnancy, and the subjective complaints are all taken into account. Since most contact lens wearers use some form of disposable lenses, which are being replaced on a regular basis anyway, it is easy to change the power of the lens temporarily.

About one in four pregnant women who wear contact lenses find their lenses become dry and uncomfortable during pregnancy. The temporary corneal swelling alters the fit and comfort of the contact lenses, so the eye doctor may refit the curvature or brand of lenses during a woman's pregnancy. Some women stop using contact lenses altogether while pregnant.

However, not all prescription shifts in pregnancy are considered normal, so it is important to let the obstetrician and eye doctor know if visual changes or blurriness occur. Diabetes and high blood pressure are both problems that sometimes arise during pregnancy. Gestational diabetes affects roughly 2 percent of pregnant women. The elevated blood sugar levels of diabetes may cause anything from minor to major internal eye bleeding, as well as swelling inside the eye, and these problems often manifest as blurry vision. Pregnancy-induced high blood pressure is called preeclampsia and may have significant consequences to the internal health of the eye. Preeclampsia also may manifest as blurry vision.

Most people are well aware that the use of tobacco products, drugs, and alcohol during pregnancy poses significant risks to the fetus. It is less well known that these substances also increase the child's risk of higher vision prescriptions, strabismus, and amblyopia. While these substances normally have addictive properties that make quitting difficult, many programs and treatment options exist. The primary care physician and obstetrician are glad to assist in smoking cessation programs.

GLAUCOMA

Glaucoma—just the word incites the fear of the unknown in most people. A 2002 Prevent Blindness America survey revealed that the top three health concerns people worried about were cancer, heart disease, and glaucoma.[12] The good news is that early detection and proper treatment can spare the eyesight of most people with the disease. Glaucoma is a group of conditions that gradually cause irreversible vision loss from optic nerve damage if left untreated. According to the World Health Organization, glaucoma is the second most common cause of blindness worldwide; cataracts are the leading cause. Nearly 2 million Americans are known to have glaucoma, and it is estimated that another 2 million have glaucoma and don't yet know it. Approximately 10 percent of people considered "legally blind" in the United States lost their sight due to glaucoma. It is not a hopeless disease, though, so continue reading.

Glaucoma is nicknamed "the sneak thief of sight" because the vision loss is gradual and typically painless. Unchecked, these "sneaky" attributes allow glaucoma to slowly decrease vision

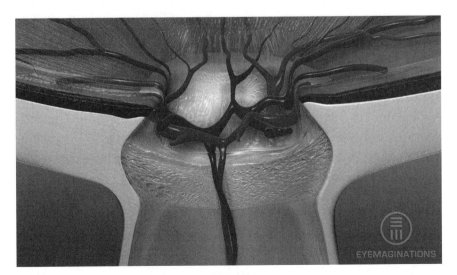

Optic Nerve Damage from Glaucoma

without detection by the individual until the loss is severe. Patients rarely schedule appointments with an eye doctor because their symptoms make them suspect they have glaucoma. *The diagnosis of glaucoma normally occurs during a comprehensive ocular health examination, rather than by a patient's vision complaints.*

Vision damage from glaucoma occurs in a slow, tunnel-vision type pattern. As the outermost peripheral vision gradually declines, it is rarely noticed by the individual until the loss is profound. The visual fields of our two eyes overlap, so if one eye has a deficiency in a particular area, the other eye usually picks up that area, making the brain still perceive vision in that area. Unless the person covers each eye alternately to test the field of vision of each eye, which most people don't routinely do, it is common to be unaware of significant visual field loss.

Self-detection of glaucoma is not influenced by socio-economic status or IQ. During my second year of practice, a new patient walked into our office and approached the front desk to schedule an appointment. He half-jokingly slammed his over-the-counter reading glasses on the desk and emphatically stated, "I can't see a darn thing with these glasses and I need to have an exam." During his examination, I discovered that this brilliant retired physics professor had lost 80 percent of the vision in each of his eyes from glaucoma. His last eye examination was over ten years prior to his visit with me, at which time he was diagnosed as mildly suspicious for glaucoma. I started him on maximum eyedrop therapy and he also underwent several glaucoma surgeries. I treated him for another ten years until he passed away. This professor lost little to no further vision after his diagnosis, but we were helpless to restore any of the massive amount of eyesight that he'd already lost.

Risk Factors for Glaucoma

Many of the risk factors for glaucoma are well known, so a person at "high risk" for glaucoma is not very difficult for an eye doctor to identify. Glaucoma affects African Americans more than any other race: it is approximately five times more prevalent in

African Americans than Caucasians; Hispanics and Asians are also at elevated risk.

Primary risk factors include African-American or Hispanic race; age of sixty years or older; family medical history of glaucoma; and history of steroid use, ocular trauma, high myopia, diabetes, or hypertension. Other risks include high eye pressure, thin corneas, history of eye injury (especially blunt trauma), and suspicious optic nerve (larger nerve center than normal).

Symptoms of Glaucoma

Glaucoma is largely symptomless, at least until the very advanced stages. However, if the pressure inside the eye is significantly elevated, you may perceive halos around lights. With substantial vision damage, there may be peripheral vision problems or tunnel vision. Individuals suffering with peripheral vision loss sometimes bump into the wall as they go around corners or complain that they don't notice cars approaching from the side and rear of their car while driving. Except in the rarest types of glaucoma, there usually is no pain associated with this condition.

Causes of Glaucoma

Glaucoma is caused by a problem with the "plumbing" of the eyes. This is an over-simplification, but in line with most of our evolving understanding about the disease. In glaucoma, the pressure inside the eyes is too high for normal tissue function, and this leads to nerve damage, specifically the nerves that carry visual information. Doctors and researchers recognize that glaucoma is likely more complicated than we have understood it to be during the last few decades. Recent research suggests that blood flow to the eyes and the optic nerve's ability to receive oxygen are also critical factors in the process of glaucoma.[13] While this may eventually lead to breakthroughs in glaucoma treatment, at this time we only have the ability to treat the internal eye pressure. Managing the intraocular pressure is, and has been, the main line of defense for decades, and today's medications are even more effective than previous generations.

The eyes produce and drain fluid inside the eye so that there is a constant fresh stream. Normally the inflow and outflow of fluid happens at equal rates, much like a faucet and a drain. The drainage mechanism in the eye is referred to as "the angle," due to the fact that several structures in the front of the eye converge, anatomically creating an angular arrangement where the fluid normally drains out. Each person's eye has a different angle width, and the width may even vary in different areas of the same eye. Larger angles are like big drain pipes, and narrower angles are like smaller drain pipes. The fluid dynamics of the eye require that it produce and drain fluid at the same rate to maintain a constant and healthy pressure within the eye. Like an overflowing sink, excess pressure in the eye may occur because the eye produces higher amounts of fluid and the drain can't keep up. Or a faulty drain may not remove fluid quickly enough, even if fluid production is normal. Either of these imbalances may cause extra fluid to build up in the eye, increasing the intraocular pressure. The delicate optic nerve, located at the back of the eye, is usually damaged

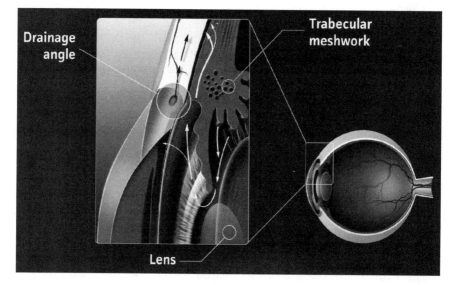

Drainage Angle of the Eye

when exposed to elevated intraocular pressure. Short intervals of increased intraocular pressure can sometimes be tolerated without permanent optic nerve damage, but sustained periods of elevated pressure over months and years is sure to cause irreversible damage. Among other jobs, the optic nerve carries visual information to the brain, so damage to this nerve means the loss of eyesight information transmitted to the brain.

Glaucoma is loosely divided into two categories: open-angle glaucoma and narrow-angle glaucoma (although there are many sub-classifications). While this chapter is not an exhaustive study on the various types of glaucoma, the information discussed here applies to most types of glaucoma.

Testing for Glaucoma

No single test allows doctors to arrive at the diagnosis of glaucoma. Multiple complex factors are considered, and the degree each risk factor plays in glaucoma is determined on an individual basis. Findings that include substantial vision loss are "cut and dried" and glaucoma treatment is commenced immediately. However, the most challenging clinical decisions are made when a patient has little or no vision loss but presents with all of the hallmark risk factors and damage may be imminent. Doctors use their knowledge and experience and the clinical findings to determine the diagnosis.

Professionals agree that a substantial "grey area" exists in the diagnosis of glaucoma. In such situations, even the patient's personal feelings about his or her existing situation may be considered in the final treatment timing decision. Some patients are very averse to any medication, and others welcome them as soon as they are considered. Clinical findings of glaucoma that are labeled normal and abnormal vary greatly from one person to another. Considering all of an individual's findings together on a case-by-case basis is a better indicator of whether glaucoma exists than comparing the at-risk patient to other glaucoma patients and their findings.

What makes the diagnosis of glaucoma elusive is that doctors are attempting to perfectly time the commencement of treatment in a small window of opportunity, and that window is rarely very clear. The perfect time to start treatment is just prior to any vision loss occurring. Initiating glaucoma treatment too early unnecessarily requires a patient to chronically use expensive prescription medications and tolerate their potential side effects for the rest of his or her life. Or, if surgery is considered, premature treatment can subject the patient to an unnecessary procedure with potentially risky complications. Conversely, if glaucoma treatment is started too late, the visual loss that has occurred is irreversible and cannot be restored, even with treatment.

So, how do doctors know when to start treatment? Fortunately, today's sophisticated computer-based instruments often allow doctors to detect "subclinical" visual changes in advance of any functional vision loss that the patient perceives. Upon detection of these early patterns of vision changes, treatment is started and the progression of vision loss is slowed, or often entirely arrested. The goal of glaucoma treatment is to halt any progressive vision loss that would have otherwise occurred without treatment. The following diagnostic findings are all considered together in the management and treatment of glaucoma.

Tonometry

Tonometry is the process of measuring the eye's internal pressure (intraocular pressure). The intraocular pressure is the fundamental measurement used in monitoring glaucoma. Abnormal elevation of intraocular pressure was once thought to be the only indicator of glaucoma, and that all high pressures equaled glaucoma. Today, intraocular pressure remains a critical piece of the diagnostic puzzle, but eye pressure is beginning to take a back seat to other findings in the overall picture. Tonometry is performed by one of various methods, all with varying degrees of accuracy and patient inconvenience. The "gold standard" method of measuring intraocular pressure in glaucoma management and treatment is called applanation tonometry. A mild anesthetic eyedrop is used to numb the eye, then a gentle probe is briefly rested on the front of the eye, painlessly obtaining an accurate measurement of the intraocular pressure.

Studies have continuously proven that high blood pressure and high intraocular pressure are *not* related or associated with each other. However, just as our blood pressure readings normally fluctuate throughout the day, our intraocular pressure is dynamic and changes throughout the day as well. Six intraocular pressure measurements spread over twelve hours will produce six different readings. The daily pressure fluctuation is normal and expected, regardless of whether glaucoma exists or not. Our intraocular pressures are at their peak around noon each day and at their lowest around 6 A.M.

Normal intraocular pressures for most people fall between 10 and 21 mmHg (measured in the same pressure scale used for blood pressure readings). The average human intraocular pressure is in the mid-teens, around 15 mmHg. Having intraocular pressure measurements above 21 mmHg doesn't necessarily mean that a person has glaucoma, but doctors may suspect possible glaucoma at that point. Tonometry is performed at each visit when a person is being monitored and treated for glaucoma, and it provides a quick and reliable way of obtaining a "snapshot" of what is happening with the disease.

High intraocular pressures permanently damage the smaller, delicate nerves that comprise the optic nerve. The optic nerve consists of millions of smaller nerves from the retina. Elevated pressures in the eye are believed to compress the nerves exiting the eye, the same way stepping on a garden hose would stop the flow of water. The compression leads to nerve death and subsequent vision loss. Intraocular pressure is the only variable we are able to control in the treatment of glaucoma, so the objective of medication and surgery is to lower the intraocular pressure so the nerves are able to continue functioning in a healthy manner. Though the processes by which glaucoma damages the eye are likely to be more complex than just pressure, scientific understanding and pharmaceutical development currently limit us to controlling only intraocular pressure. This treatment approach to glaucoma management has proven successful over the last few decades.

Opthalmoscopy

Ophthalmoscopy is the process of imaging and studying the retina and optic nerve. Various handheld instruments, lenses, head loupes, and laser scanners aid the doctor in the study of the internal eye. The optic nerve and its anatomic appearance vary slightly in each person, just like fingerprints. Doctors evaluate each optic nerve and compare their findings to the established ranges of normal and abnormal appearances. A specific measurement called the "cup-to-disc" ratio is determined and recorded for each patient. The cup-to-disc norms vary between groups of differing ethnic origins, and even between individuals of the same race. Similar to intraocular pressures, the medical community has identified a standard range of normal optic nerve appearances, but they are never absolute. Thus, individuals with optic nerves considered to be in the normal ranges can still unquestionably suffer from vision loss due to glaucoma. Likewise, many individuals with optic nerves considered to have an abnormal "glaucoma-like" appearance can have perfectly functioning vision with no degradation over time.

A healthy optic nerve should not change appearance in an individual over the course of his or her lifetime. However, a patient suffering from glaucoma has nerve dropout (cellular death in the optic nerve), which slowly changes the anatomic appearance of the optic nerve over time. This slow change is challenging, but not impossible, for an eye doctor to observe, and highly sophisticated and accurate retinal scanning lasers are able to image minute changes. Laser scanners can alert the doctor of harmful changes occurring to the optic nerve years in advance of what direct observations would detect.

Perimetry

Perimetry (measurement of the "visual field") is the assessment and record of what each eye is able to see centrally and peripherally. A visual field test produces a map of the eye's ability and sensitivity levels in all areas of its field of view. Databases of normal and abnormal degrees of visual field in all directions around the line of sight, as well as their relative sensitivities, are compared with

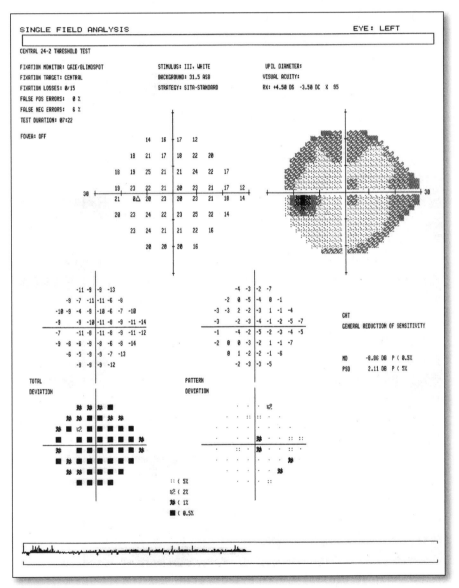

Visual Field Test

the patient's results to help identify areas of abnormality. Though visual fields were once measured manually, computers now obtain very sensitive and reliable information about a person's field of view and relative brightness sensitivities. There are recognizable patterns of visual field loss in glaucoma, and computerized visual field instruments are sensitive enough (via the doctor's interpretation) to detect these early patterns of vision loss.

Even though laser scans of the optic nerve can detect patterns of loss earlier than visual fields can, some doctors feel the results from perimetry are more concrete and reliable. All pieces of data need to be considered along with several other findings. Perimetry is used continuously in the management of glaucoma to determine if the visual field is changing. Stable visual fields are the objective, and the test is repeated from every few months to once a year, depending on the status of the condition being monitored.

Central Corneal Thickness

It wasn't until 2002 that the central corneal thickness (CCT) measurement was added as a vital piece of information routinely assessed for glaucoma patients. A landmark study showed that the thickness of an individual's cornea affects the accuracy of eye pressure measurements.[14] When testing the intraocular pressure, the probe from the tonometer gently rests on the central cornea. It is now understood that an adjustment to the intraocular pressure measurements needs to be made based on the thickness of the individual's cornea. A patient with a thicker-than-average cornea falsely reads higher than the true pressure, while a patient with a thinner-than-average cornea falsely reads lower. Today, doctors adjust the clinical intraocular pressure readings accordingly, based on the patient's corneal thickness.

Central corneal thickness is measured in a method similar to tonometry using a painless, ultrasonic probe. Unless laser refractive surgery is performed, it is rare for someone's corneal thickness to change over time. For this reason, central corneal thickness only needs to be measured once or twice over a lifetime.

Gonioscopy

Gonioscopy is the clinical test used to view the fluid drainage mechanism of the eye (the "angle"). Constantly regenerated fluid needs to drain out of the eye at the same rate that it is produced to maintain a healthy balance of internal fluid and intraocular pressure. Since the part of the eye that drains the fluid can't be viewed directly with a microscope, a special mirrored lens allows doctors to see around the corners of the eye to view the drainage mechanism. The gonioscopy lens is a large contact lens gently placed on an anesthetized eye for less than two minutes, allowing the doctor to determine the size of the drainage mechanism, as well as to see if there is any debris blocking it. Loose pigment, debris from ocular trauma, abnormal blood vessel growth, and even tumors can block the drainage mechanism. Laser treatments of the drainage mechanism, if necessary, are delivered to the angle through the gonioscopy lens as well.

Treatment of Glaucoma

Once the decision to treat glaucoma is made, a number of tools are available to control the disease. Prescription eyedrops are the primary way glaucoma is managed. Intraocular pressure–reducing medications slow down or stop optic nerve damage that leads to vision loss. These medications won't reverse any vision loss that has already occurred, but they may prevent further loss. There are dozens of prescription eyedrops available, and they each work through different means to achieve the same outcome. Some work to slow down the eye's ability to produce fluid, and others work by increasing the rate of fluid drainage out of the eye (several prescriptions combine two drugs that use both methods).

Older drugs such as Timolol have been successfully used since the 1970s and are at times still used today. While these medications worked with great efficacy, some carried undesirable side effects, particularly for those with existing heart and lung conditions. Today's glaucoma eyedrops are typically more effective, require lower doses, and carry fewer side effects.

A classification of glaucoma drugs called "prostaglandin analogs" are typically the first line of defense against glaucoma, though not all patients or types of glaucoma respond well to this drug class. Xalatan, Travatan, and Lumigan are the three most frequently prescribed drugs in this class. Potential side effects include burning, redness of the eyes, thickening and darkening of the eyelashes, and darkening of the iris color in patients with lighter-colored eyes. Often, the burning subsides after a few weeks of use; the eyelash thickening may be pronounced, but switching to another medication will usually reverse the lash growth.

The doctor will closely follow the patient to monitor the pressure-lowering effects of these medications. Many doctors set a custom "target pressure" for each patient at the onset of treatment, which takes into account multiple factors. Reaching the target pressure may occur with a single medication, with a combination of drugs, or may even include surgery as part of the plan, depending on the particular case.

The eyedrops for glaucoma work only while they are being taken as prescribed. It is a lifetime therapy, much like treating hypertension. Compliance can be difficult and the medications may be costly. I'll sometimes hear patients say, "These drops don't seem to do anything" or, "My vision doesn't seem any different with these drops." Indeed, glaucoma medications do not make vision better, but they are the best insurance that symptoms don't get worse. Helping you see the same each day is exactly what they are designed to do.

If eyedrop compliance is difficult, or the treatment simply doesn't achieve the target pressures, glaucoma surgery is an option. The most common laser procedures—argon laser trebeculoplasty (ALT) and selective laser trebeculoplasty (SLT)—use lasers to facilitate the fluid drainage from the eye. Glaucoma laser surgery is a relatively painless and quick, and it can profoundly improve the control of glaucoma. However, the results are variable depending on the type of glaucoma and the patient's eye anatomy, and laser surgery will sometimes lose its effect after a few years, so the eye may need to be treated again.

Older, more conventional forms of glaucoma surgery are still useful today, particularly for very aggressive and advanced forms of the disease. Some surgeries alter the eye's drainage mechanism without the use of lasers; for example, a small tube can be surgically inserted into the eye to help drain excess fluid.

Given the common fear about getting glaucoma, and the significant quality-of-life issue that vision loss would entail, the best advice I can render is to make sure that you have an eye examination every year or two at minimum, even if you have no eye problems or don't wear glasses. During a comprehensive ocular exam, your eye doctor will spend as much time assessing the overall health of your eyes as he or she does your vision. Early detection of glaucoma is essential for preservation of eyesight, and regular eye examinations will stop this terrible eye disease in its tracks before it can do serious damage.

KERATOCONUS

Keratoconus is a condition characterized by a progressive deformation of the cornea. The irregular corneal shape distorts the optics of the eye similar to the way a warped eyeglass lens would. Rather than exhibiting the smooth curvature expected of a healthy cornea, the eye develops variable areas of steepening throughout the tissue. Keratoconus varies in severity among individuals, ranging from very mild to extreme visual distortion. It typically affects both eyes, but in an asymmetric fashion—one eye is nearly always warped and "cone shaped" more severely than the other.

The corneal warpage is often first diagnosed in adolescence and usually plateaus in severity in the person's twenties and thirties. Though not fully understood, it is believed to be genetically related. Affecting approximately one out of every 1,000 people, there appears to be no predilection for a particular race or gender. Once diagnosed, the course of the condition is quite unpredictable.

While keratoconus may cause nothing more than a minute, bland distortion that is nearly without bother to the individual, in the majority of cases the visual distortion ultimately requires the use of specialized rigid gas permeable contact lenses (RGPs). RGPs effectively compensate for the corneal warpage, allowing the individual to lead a normal life. In severe cases, the corneal warpage may progress beyond even what RGPs can address and corneal transplantation may be required.

Symptoms of Keratoconus

The initial symptoms of keratoconus begin innocuously, necessitating more frequent updates to eyeglass prescriptions. Visual distortion, multiple images, ghosting, glare, and light sensitivity gradually increase while the rate and severity of eyeglass prescription updates accelerate over months or years. Most prescription changes related to keratoconus primarily affect the astigmatism component. Even if large shifts in astigmatism don't alert the eye doctor to the possibility of early keratoconus, the inability to get an eye to see 20/20 with the updated prescription may be another red flag. As the cornea distorts, eyeglasses no longer fully compensate for the visually deforming effects.

Eye doctors are familiar with the early signs of keratoconus and will measure the shape of the cornea using corneal topography. Like a topographical relief map, computerized corneal topography instruments map the elevations and shape of the cornea, making the diagnosis of keratoconus fairly straightforward. Except in rare cases of corneal hydrops (the most severe form of keratoconus), it is usually a painless condition.

Causes of Keratoconus

Though well studied, the cause of keratoconus is still unknown. It is surmised that an autosomal dominant genetic pattern exists in its inheritance pattern. Not all children of a parent with keratoconus will develop the condition themselves. Associations with certain types of allergies, and rubbing the eyes vigorously, have been implicated as potential causes. Individuals with Down syndrome are known to have a higher incidence of keratoconus.

Treatment of Keratoconus

In the early stages of keratoconus, frequent updates to the eyeglass or soft contact lens prescription simply keep pace with the developing corneal changes. Unfortunately, though, most patients eventually reach a stage where the eyeglasses no longer entirely compensate for the visual problems, and RGPs need to be used. RGPs rest directly on the cornea, effectively "smoothing out" the irregular shape and usually restoring good optical quality. Many keratoconic patients unable to obtain 20/20 vision with eyeglasses do achieve it with RGPs. If corneal warpage continues to progress, more customized and complicated rigid contact lens designs can help keratoconus patients maintain clear eyesight.

Approximately 15–20 percent of people affected by keratoconus suffer from continual degradation of eyesight, even with the use of RGPs. In the most severe cases, a corneal transplant is the last remaining measure to potentially restore eyesight. After a donor cornea is located, a surgeon creates a "button" of the distorted corneal tissue, removes it, and grafts normal donor tissue in its place. The success rate of corneal transplantation for the treatment of keratoconus is high, but it is not guaranteed.

A newer treatment that shows promise is the use of segmented intrastromal corneal rings. Made of materials similar to contact lenses, these half-circle shaped rings are surgically inserted into the cornea around the line of sight. The rings act to stabilize the cornea and help regulate the shape abnormalities that cause visual distortions. (The brand name of the corneal rings is Intacs, Addition Technology, Inc., Sunnyvale, CA; www.intacsforkeratoconus.com.)

EYELID TWITCHING

Eyelid twitches are involuntary, annoying muscle spasms of the eyelids that seem to appear out of nowhere. These episodes of "eyelid jumping" typically affect the lower eyelids more than the upper ones, and they are fairly common. Though it feels like the entire eye is shaking, the lid twitch is rarely noticeable to anyone other than the affected person. Lid twitching may last a few hours, days, weeks, or even months before resolving.

The most common cause of eyelid twitching is stress. No part of our body is immune from the effects of stress, and an eyelid twitch is one of the primary ocular manifestations. It is not uncommon for the twitch to begin several weeks after a particularly stressful time or event, even if it feels like the stress has passed. Emotional stress, physical stress, and lack of sleep are common triggers for eyelid twitches. Other potential causes include excess caffeine or alcohol consumption, seasonal allergies, and potassium or magnesium deficiencies.

Taking a multivitamin supplement may help resolve an active lid twitch. In rare but severe cases of lid twitching, Botox® treatments effectively interrupt and stop the twitching episode. Eyelid twitches are normally harmless and have no long-term ocular health implications, and most cases eventually resolve by themselves and require no treatment. However, eyelid twitches that also involve the facial muscles, last longer than one week, or include a droopy eyelid should be medically evaluated by a physician or eye doctor, since they may indicate a more serious underlying neurological condition.

CHAPTER 8

SENIOR EYE ISSUES

Though conditions such as dry eye syndrome, glaucoma, and eye infections have already been addressed in the chapters about eye issues affecting children and adults, these and other problems may affect seniors as well. This chapter specifically addresses cataracts and macular degeneration, conditions normally associated with seniors. Cataracts may occur at any age, though their prevalence increases with age. Macular degeneration typically manifests in individuals sixty-five and older. While cataracts and macular degeneration are caused by multiple factors, it is interesting to note that ultraviolet exposure (over the course of a lifetime) is thought to play a substantial role in the cause of each condition.

CATARACTS

The physiological lens in the eye is an amazing optical structure. At birth, this lens is a clear and flexible tissue that rapidly changes shape to adapt to the eye's focusing needs from second to second. The lens is comprised mostly of water and protein, and the proteins are arranged in such an organized manner that the result is a transparent tissue that allows light to pass through. The "ravages of time" change our skin and the lenses in our eyes in much the same way. With maturity, the once smooth and supple skin begins to wrinkle and change color. Similarly, the lens in each eye gradually hardens and becomes less clear with age. A cataract causes a decline in eyesight due to clouding and distortion of the previously clear lens. Everyone suffers from cataracts to some degree if they live long enough, but at what age and how much cataracts affect each person varies. Several external factors affect the timeline, but cataracts are about as inevitable as the aging process itself. Fortunately, the reduced vision from cataracts is treatable, usually restoring the clarity of our eyesight to that of youth.

In describing cataracts to patients, I compare them to a dirty windshield in a car. The windshield may be dirty and obscured over the entire surface, or there may be some areas that are perfectly clear while others are dirty. There may even be "stars" in the glass due to rock chips. The location of windshield dirt governs how much it affects a driver's vision. If a large area of dirt is only over the passenger side of the windshield, the dirt is not likely to hinder the driver much. However, if the entire windshield is clean with the exception of a small area right in front of the driver's line of sight, that area of dirt may significantly impede the driver's ability to see well. Cataracts affect our eyesight in much the same way: some types of cataracts cloud the whole physiological lens equally, and other types obscure only very specific areas.

Types of Cataracts

The most common type of cataracts are called nuclear cataracts, in which an equally distributed yellow haze affects the entire area of the lens. Like automobile headlights that become hazy and discolored over time, nuclear lens changes usually occur slowly and the onset of symptoms is gradual. Eventually, the yellowish hazing of the lens becomes so dense that the individual complains of a chronic film or haze to their eyesight.

Cortical cataracts are usually denser and more opaque than nuclear cataracts. On the other hand, cortical cataracts start off affecting a smaller area of the overall lens. Cortical cataracts frequently appear in the shape of a piece of pie. As cortical lens changes progress, the size of the "pie piece" gets larger. Cortical cataracts are normally widest at the outside of the lens and come to a point near the center of the lens. Patients become very symptomatic once the tips of the "pie pieces" reach the center of the lens.

Posterior subcapsular cataracts (PSCs) are opacifications that obscure the central back side of the lens. Posterior subcapsular cataracts are often associated with the use of steroid medications, but that is not always the case. Even a small PSC may potentially cause big vision problems until it is removed. This type of cataract can dramatically degrade vision in a very short period of time. Some patients with PSCs go from having no symptoms to significant visual changes in a matter of weeks.

Nuclear, cortical, and posterior subcapsular cataracts are the three most common types of cataracts. Though the manner in which each type of cataract affects vision is slightly different, their treatment is the same. Entire textbooks have been written to exhaustively cover the various types of cataracts that exist, but the fundamental problem of any cataract is that it interferes with the clear transmission of light to the retina.

Risk Factors for Cataracts

Just as dermatologists remind us to protect our skin from the sun's ultraviolet (UV) rays by using sunscreen, protecting our eyes from UV light is just as important. Ultraviolet light is believed to be the primary cause of cataracts for most people. UV light exposure is received when we are in sunlight, so we need to limit our UV exposure. However, the body uses ultraviolet light to synthesize vitamin D, so completely eliminating UV exposure is not recommended.

Farmers, lifeguards, "sun-worshipers," and those living near the equator are all groups that demonstrate an increased incidence and earlier onset of cataracts. It is sensible to use 100 percent UV blocking sunglasses when outdoors. A great deal of UV damage done to the eyes occurs prior to age eighteen, precisely the age group least likely to wear sunglasses. While African-Americans are less prone to UV skin damage than Caucasians, they are still just as susceptible to cataracts from UV light and should be equally concerned about protecting their eyes.

Other risk factors for cataracts include diabetes, smoking, trauma to the eye, electrocution, and prolonged steroid use. Steroids such as prednisone are commonly prescribed to treat conditions such as arthritis, asthma, and other autoimmune diseases. Using steroids for a few days or weeks poses little increased risk, but long-term usage at higher doses is strongly linked to cataract formation. Cataracts may also form as a result of ocular trauma. Traumatic cataracts may not develop until long after the initial injury; people with a history of "black eyes" or sports injuries, as well as car accident victims who have suffered head trauma, sometimes develop cataracts months or years later.

Symptoms of Cataracts

The symptoms vary according to the type of cataract but commonly include complaints of cloudiness to the vision as well as an overall reduction of the best corrected vision. Many describe it as a constant "film" or "skim" over the vision that won't go away.

Additionally, increased glare is among the top complaints caused by cataracts. Glare is typically most bothersome at night, especially while driving. The cataract opacities in the lens act to scatter light entering the eyes, inducing glare. The glare and scattered light may be so pronounced that they cause double vision. Cataracts often cause colors to lose their vibrancy, and people complain that colors become "washed out." The color vision changes are gradual, so they may not be perceived until the cataract is removed, upon which color vision quickly restores to normal.

Frequent changes to the eyeglass prescription are common as cataracts are developing, sometimes requiring a change in lenses two or three times per year. Physiologically, the lens inside the eye thickens as a result of cataracts. The lens thickening simultane-

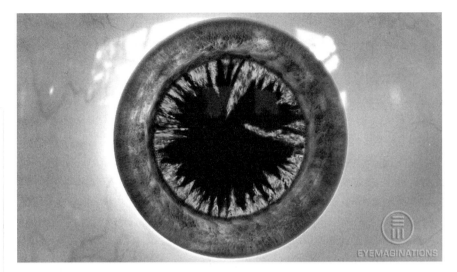

Cortical Cataracts

ously changes the eye's ability to focus light, which requires a corresponding change to the eyeglass prescription.

Reduced vision from cataracts affects different people to varying degrees. A cataract that allows an individual to see no better than 20/30 may not hinder some people at all, while others complain that they are unable to be functional at this level of vision. The explanation for the variation in complaints is twofold. The first is lifestyle: someone regularly performing visually demanding tasks such as trying to read stock quotes, working crossword puzzles, or sewing will find cataracts to be more troublesome than someone who requires their eyesight to perform less demanding work. Secondly, each person has a different visual threshold: by nature, some people require sharper eyesight than others, just as each person has a different pain tolerance level to the same stimulus.

Testing for Cataracts

Specialized testing to diagnose a cataract is minimal. Arguably, the most difficult part of a cataract diagnosis is ruling out other coexisting alternate causes of reduced vision that may be present in addition to the cataract. A cataract is easily recognizable to the eye doctor during a microscopic examination of the eyes, and some cataracts are so advanced they may be diagnosed without the use of a microscope.

Normal eyeglass prescription changes still occur as they did prior to the formation of cataracts, and other sight-threatening conditions such as macular degeneration and glaucoma may co-exist with cataracts. What percentage of vision reduction is due to cataracts versus other underlying conditions is challenging, if not impossible, for a doctor to determine. The only way to accurately determine the answer is to remove one of the known causes and evaluate the remaining source in isolation. Often, diseases that occur simultaneously with cataracts can't be removed, but the cataracts can be. An instrument called a potential acuity meter (PAM) may assist the doctor in estimating the potential visual acuity after cataract surgery. Doctors and surgeons want to assure a patient considering surgery to the best of their ability and want the surgery to actually result in improved eyesight. If the reduced eyesight thought to be from cataracts were actually attributable to some other underlying condition, there may be no improvement in eyesight after cataract surgery. This outcome is disappointing and frustrating to everyone involved.

Testing for cataracts involves an analysis of the patient's symptoms and the best corrected visual acuity after an updated prescription, as well as physical observation of the lens through a dilated pupil. The doctor's evaluation of this data typically results in a reliable cataract diagnosis. The question that follows an initial cataract diagnosis is, "What should I do about it?"

Treatment of Cataracts

Early stages of cataracts are managed without surgery. Updating eyeglass lenses to keep pace with the changes induced by cataracts is critical. Often small changes to an eyeglass prescription can significantly optimize eyesight prior to the patient requiring surgery.

It is not unusual to need eyeglass prescription updates more frequently in the early stages of cataract development. Non-glare lens treatments for the eyeglass lenses help reduce (but do not eliminate) glare caused by the cataracts.

The cataract's opacification of the lens filters the amount of incoming light reaching the retina. Increasing the level of ambient light is universally beneficial for cataract patients, especially when reading. By pointing a light source directly at the reading material, reading requires less effort. While increasing light is helpful, in some ways it is also a hindrance: since cataracts scatter light, increased levels of light creates more glare. Most patients still prefer having the added light levels, even if it does increase glare.

One of the best ways of optimizing vision with cataracts is to use prescription polarized sunglasses while outside and when driving. Polarized lenses filter out light rays that contribute to glare, and they effectively counteract glare caused by cataracts by reducing the light scatter. While many sunglass companies claim that certain colored tints on the lenses help improve vision with cataracts, no tints of any specific color have been definitively shown to help cataract patients. The decision regarding colored tints often comes down to personal preference of which color "feels" the best to the individual. In my experience, it's best to avoid colored tints and stick with brown or grey polarized lenses when trying to enhance eyesight affected by cataracts.

Updated eyeglass prescriptions and polarized lenses will help for only so long, and then the cataracts usually progress to the point at which glasses no longer improve vision. This is when the doctor will begin talking about considering cataract surgery.

Surgery is the definitive solution to cataracts, but not all cataracts require surgery immediately, and some cataracts never require surgery. The point at which a cataract requires surgery is more heavily influenced by the patient's informed decision than it is the doctor telling the patient they must undergo the surgery. The benefits begin to outweigh the risks of cataract surgery in the ranges of 20/30 to 20/40 best corrected vision or worse. Lifestyle is a large factor in determining the appropriate time for surgery. If an individual is still able to drive safely (determined by the doctor, not the patient!) and perform daily functions without complaint, often surgery will be delayed. If the reduced vision from cataracts affects one's lifestyle so much that they can't participate in the activities they enjoy, then cataract surgery should be considered. For many people, the thought of surgery is unimaginable and they subsequently decide that they'd rather live with the poor vision in lieu of undergoing surgery. It is a personal choice and the doctor will respect your decision either way. I normally encourage patients to pursue surgery when indicated since the eyesight is so dramatically improved in nearly all cases. It should be noted that allowing cataracts to progress to very advanced stages prior to having surgery makes good surgical outcomes more difficult to obtain.

Surgery of any kind is a major consideration, but fortunately cataract surgery is less risky than most other types of surgery. Cataract removal surgery is the most commonly performed surgical procedure in the United States, and most surgeons have well-honed skills with this procedure. The majority of patients have cataract surgery on an outpatient basis, so an overnight hospital stay is not required. However, the patient's overall physical health is a large factor in determining the ease or difficulty with which the surgery is performed. Patients with uncontrolled diabetes or other unstable conditions that compromise their health and healing capability may require overnight observation at a hospital when having cataracts removed.

If cataract surgery is required in both eyes, the eye with the most advanced cataract will be treated with the initial surgery. A second surgery for the other eye is then scheduled one to two months afterward. Unless it's an emergency, cataract surgery is rarely performed on both eyes during the same day. Though surgical risks are low, the benefit of delaying the second surgery outweighs the small risk of an unexpected complication affecting both eyes during the same procedure. Should something rare and unfortunate happen, such as an uncontrollable post-operative infection, the risk is limited to only one eye.

Two types of cataract surgery are commonly performed today. The most common type is called phacoemulsification, but extracapsular extraction is still used as well, depending on the surgeon and the type of cataract to be removed. Uncomplicated cataract surgery usually takes a surgeon 15–20 minutes to perform and is painless for the patient since local anesthesia of the eye is used. The patient is awake during the surgery and is not exposed to the additional risks that general anesthesia carries. If the patient desires, the doctor is able to talk with the patient about what is happening during the procedure. A small, precisely placed incision is made in the eye at the onset of surgery. (Phacoemulsification surgery requires a smaller incision than extracapsular extraction.) After the incision is made, the surgeon removes the cloudy cataract lens and cleans the surrounding tissue as needed. Then, an artificial intraocular lens (IOL) is inserted.

The IOL is like a small internal contact lens that rarely needs to be removed or reinserted again after the initial surgery. These implantable lenses are fabricated with prescriptions for nearsightedness, farsightedness, astigmatism, or even multifocal uses. A lens implant prescription calculation is made for each eye prior to surgery, although it is challenging to predict the exact prescription needed in advance because the cataract interferes with a precise measurement. However, the IOLs allow the surgeon to sometimes completely compensate for the vision prescription that existed before surgery.

Most intraocular lenses are single vision, which means they correct the distance vision only. Reading glasses are still likely necessary after cataract surgery. More sophisticated ways of dealing with multiple prescriptions do exist. Some patients elect to have monovision IOLs so that the implant in one eye is focused for the distance and the other eye's implant is focused for reading. Another option is a multifocal IOL, which has the ability to focus distance and near images, though not perfectly. While these are more expensive, they typically give you the ability to see reasonably well at all distances without the use of eyeglasses. Reading glasses may still be needed occasionally in addition to the multifocal IOLs. Not all prescriptions are compatible with multi-focal IOLs; a further consideration is whether or not you are willing to accept the slight blurriness that occurs with these lenses.

When the surgery is complete, some surgeons tape an eye patch over the eye. A shield "goggle" is worn at night so that the patient does not accidentally rub the eye during sleep. The eye patch is removed at the one-day follow-up examination, and often an immediate improvement in vision is noticed. The eye will be blood-shot and have considerable swelling the day after the surgery; this is normal in the beginning and will resolve after a few days or weeks. After surgery, the vision generally continues to improve in the first week as the swelling reduces. The surgeon prescribes a regimen of prescription eyedrops to use for infection prevention, reduction of inflammation, and to control any discomfort.

Side effects as a result of cataract surgery are rare, and cataracts don't come back once they've been removed. However, the most common side effect of cataract surgery is the development of what's referred to as an "after-cataract" or posterior capsular opacification. During cataract surgery, the lens is removed from a sack-like tissue called the capsule. The surgeon then clears the capsule of any remaining debris and the intraocular lens is placed in the remaining capsule. If even just a few invisible capsular cells are left behind, they may grow and cause a film over the back surface of the implanted lens. This film appears after approximately 20 percent of cataract surgeries. Fortunately, it is fairly easy to fix the "after-cataract" with in-office laser surgery. Less common side effects of cataract surgery include a droopy eyelid or increased intraocular pressures. Additionally, chronic swelling of the cornea and retina may sometimes occur, but these are usually treatable conditions. The doctor will monitor for the development of post-operative complications during follow-up visits.

Ophthalmologists who operate on cataracts are easy to find

unless you live in a rural area. Friends who have already undergone cataract surgery are good referral sources for finding a surgeon. Another option is your optometrist: since your optometrist won't be the one performing the operation and has seen the results of many local surgeons, they can be an excellent, unbiased resource for cataract surgery referral.

MACULAR DEGENERATION

Age-related macular degeneration (AMD) is a foreboding diagnosis because it is a challenging disease to live with. While progress has been made, the medical treatments available for AMD do not universally prevent vision loss. Macular degeneration is the leading cause of blindness in Americans over sixty-five years old, the number one threat to eyesight as we mature. Approximately 200,000 new cases of macular degeneration are diagnosed in the United States each year, which in total affects about 15 million Americans. The silver lining to this is that scientists are aggressively researching macular degeneration and treatments are evolving at a rapid pace. I firmly hope and believe that we will find a cure for macular degeneration. Plus, many of the factors that contribute to the development of macular degeneration are modifiable behaviors, so you can lower your risk of developing the condition.

Types of Macular Degeneration

"Dry" and "wet" macular degeneration are the two types of AMD. Dry macular degeneration is also known as non-exudative or non-neovascular macular degeneration, and it is the first phase of the disease. Approximately 10 percent of the people with dry macular degeneration progress to the more serious stage of the disease called wet macular degeneration (sometimes referred to as exudative or neovascular macular degeneration).

The macula, or fovea, is a specific area of the retina in each eye that measures about 1 mm in diameter. The macula is responsible for a large percentage of eyesight—namely, the central vision. If your field of vision had crosshairs (like the center of a camera viewfinder), the macula would be responsible for the central area of eyesight where the crosshairs intersect. Having the highest resolution of the entire retina, the macula provides the part of the vision that is used to look directly at something. Because the macula is responsible for such high visual detail, it has a very dense concentration of cells with a correspondingly rich blood supply to feed all of the cells.

In AMD, some or all of the macular cells degenerate and die. As these cells "drop out," the corresponding parts of the eyesight they're responsible for no longer register vision. Though AMD takes away from the central vision, the good news is that no one goes entirely blind from this disease. A person with AMD loses the ability to gaze directly at a visual target, but they can still perceive movement and vision in a circular area outside of the lost central vision (peripheral vision). Coping methods such as "eccentric fixation" can be learned to help work around the visual limitations. Eccentric fixation is the process of directing the eyesight off to the side of the intended visual target. AMD patients often can't read

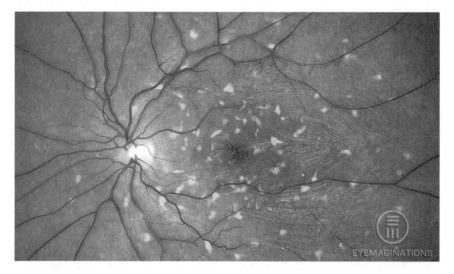

Dry Macular Degeneration

certain letters on an eye chart when asked to look at them directly, but if they "point" their vision one or two letters to the left or right of the target, their peripheral vision often sees the intended object.

Dry macular degeneration is often signaled to the doctor by the presence of *drusen* in or around the macula. Drusen are small, yellowish retinal deposits that may occur from the leftover debris of cellular breakdown and metabolism. Drusen deposits found outside of the macula are generally harmless and have no effect on vision. However, drusen in the macular area disrupt the normal organization and functioning of the macular cells and possibly indicate impending progressive macular degeneration.

Wet macular degeneration is the combination of dry AMD plus the growth of new, unwanted blood vessels in the macula. The body thinks that it needs to supply more oxygen to the areas of the macula that have died, so it compensates by growing new blood vessels (neo-vascularization) in the macular area. The additional oxygen supply from these vessels is seemingly helpful, but in actuality it is harmful. The new blood vessels are weak and have a tendency to leak blood and component fluids. When one or more of

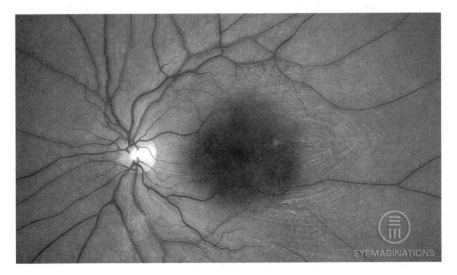

Wet Macular Degeneration

these fragile new vessels ruptures, spilling blood into the macula, the effect on the eyesight is devastating. Blood in undesired areas of the retina obscures eyesight wherever it goes.

Risk Factors for Macular Degeneration

The exact causes and origins of macular degeneration are not yet fully understood; nonetheless, there is a great deal we do know about it. The two largest factors believed to contribute to the formation of AMD are age and a family history of the disease. Macular degeneration is well known to be more prevalent with aging, and a genetic predisposition to AMD exists with a family history of its presence in one or both parents. Women are at slightly higher risk than men, and Caucasians are thought to be at moderately higher risk for developing AMD than a more darkly pigmented individual (but all races are affected).

A few environmental factors are thought to play a role in the development of macular degeneration. Cigarette smoking is known to increase the incidence of macular degeneration, and a possible association between UV light exposure and macular degeneration exists, too. Both UV exposure and cigarette smoking are modifiable factors and changing behaviors can help reduce the chance of developing this potentially debilitating ocular disease.

The strong association between smoking cigarettes and the incidence of macular degeneration is known to be a major factor in developing this sight-robbing disease, though it is not the only cause. Quitting the habit of smoking is challenging to accomplish, but it is possible with assistance. The health benefits gained from a smoking cessation program reach far beyond the eyes, as we know. As in cataracts, people with high UV exposure over the course of their lives seem to demonstrate a higher incidence of macular degeneration. Studies have not as strongly associated UV exposure with AMD as with smoking, but protecting our eyes from UV light has greater benefits beyond potentially preventing AMD. Since ultraviolet light is implicated in cataracts and various skin cancers (frequently around the eyes and eyelids), protecting the eyes from

UV light is still beneficial, whether it is eventually proven to be linked to macular degeneration or not. Much of the damage to the eyes from UV light occurs before the age of eighteen, so a childhood history of UV exposure is potentially a greater risk factor than UV exposure as an adult. Still, limiting UV exposure and using high-quality 100 percent UV blocking sunglasses when outdoors are habits that are beneficial and easy to adopt.

Diet is also believed to play a role in macular degeneration, but considerable debate exists as to what dietary components play the biggest roles. The oxidative processes in our body's cells are factors in the aging process, and antioxidants are believed to have protective roles in the macula and other parts of the body. Antioxidants are nutrients that can be obtained through the diet or supplementation. Many vegetables are rich in antioxidants, particularly the green leafy vegetables such as spinach and kale. Additionally, yellow and orange squashes contain antioxidants and should be consumed in abundance. Vitamin supplements are discussed in more detail later in this chapter under "Treatment for Macular Degeneration."

Symptoms of Macular Degeneration

The symptoms of macular degeneration often emerge gradually. AMD typically affects both eyes, but in an asymmetric fashion; one eye is usually further advanced than the other. Early symptoms of AMD include mild to moderate loss of central visual acuity, which does not fully improve with new eyeglasses. Prior to a diagnosis of AMD, most people assume this blurriness is the result of an outdated eyeglass prescription or early cataracts. When the newly updated eyeglass prescription fails to restore vision to 20/20, the doctor will suspect an underlying problem such as macular degeneration and investigate further. An examination of the inside of the eye through a dilated pupil will allow the doctor to observe the signs of AMD when they are present.

People with macular degeneration require more light than normal to see well. As dry AMD progresses, the lowest readable line on the eye chart gradually increases in size up the chart as acuity is affected. Currently, there are no *surgical* treatments that can intervene with the progressive visual loss associated with dry macular degeneration. As discussed earlier, lifestyle modifications can be extremely helpful at this stage.

As eyesight declines, a continuous and bothersome blurry central area directly in the line of sight emerges. At this stage, people find that they no longer receive visual information by looking directly at an object. However, they learn that they can still receive some eyesight by looking to the side of the object, thus utilizing the intact peripheral vision.

Symptoms of wavy or distorted images in the central part of the eyesight may be an early sign that wet macular degeneration is impending. It is critical that any newly detected waviness or changes in distortion are reported to the eye doctor immediately. There is a small window of time in which doctors can intervene surgically to prevent further impending catastrophic vision loss. Waviness often indicates early leaking of the new blood vessel growth in the macular area. If one of the new vessels spills blood, an acute and significant further reduction of vision occurs.

Eye doctors often instruct patients to self-test each eye at home on a regular basis for new symptoms of this central waviness. A simple black-and-white grid called an Amsler Grid (see page 161) can be used for self-monitoring of central waviness.

Testing for Macular Degeneration

Signs and symptoms are evaluated together in the diagnosis of macular degeneration. Signs that doctors observe include reduced visual acuity through new eyeglasses, as well as physiological changes observed in the macula as examined through a dilated pupil. Macular degeneration varies in presentation from one person to another, but it is characteristically recognizable to an eye doctor during a thorough exam of the retina. Macular degeneration is usually progressive and each subsequent exam of the macula may yield a slightly different appearance. Documentation

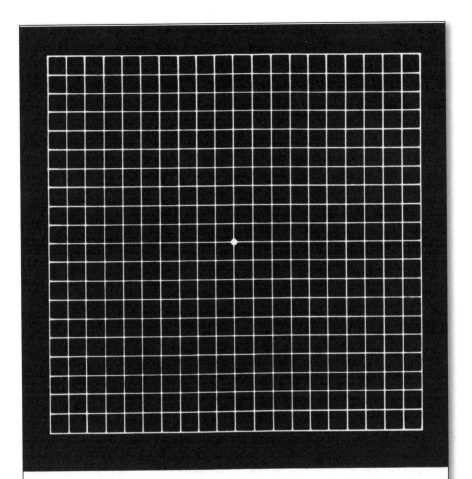

GENERAL INSTRUCTIONS

- Card should be held 12 inches from eyes.

- Test the right eye first by covering the left eye. Repeat procedure on the left eye by covering the right eye.

- Concentrate on the center dot, noticing any waves, distortions, or blind spots in the lines. If problems are noticed, inform your vision-care specialist immeditely.

Amsler Grid

of the macula with photographs better allow doctors to monitor the rate of progression. In addition, photography helps gauge whether the dry form is converting to the wet form of AMD.

A decade ago, doctors relied on their own eyes and fluorescein-dye testing to determine whether the small blood vessels were growing in the macula. Though dry AMD is not surgically treatable, new blood vessel growth can be surgically treated in hopes of preventing a major bleed in the macula. Doctors vigilantly watch for these harmful blood vessels and surgeons immediately attempt to eliminate them when detected. Surgery doesn't cure AMD, but in many cases it prevents further damage. Today's ocular examination technology is amazing. Fluoroscein-dye testing and advanced scanning lasers aid in the evaluation of the macula to detect microscopic changes that are measured in microns. The retinal scanning laser technology used today gives advanced warning of impending and treatable changes in macular degeneration. This warning now comes far earlier than technology afforded doctors just a few years ago.

Treatment for Macular Degeneration

There is no cure for age-related macular degeneration, but treatments can sometimes help diminish the negative effects and delay the progression of disease. Many treatments help prolong intact eyesight. Treatment for macular degeneration can be divided into two categories, surgical and nonsurgical.

Nonsurgical treatments include some easily modifiable lifestyle factors. If it is not already a habit, patients diagnosed with macular degeneration should protect their eyes against UV rays with high-quality sunglasses. The UV protection does not need to be used indoors, but should be used all daytime hours spent outdoors and while driving during the day. Because ultraviolet rays from the sun are not entirely blocked by clouds, it is possible to get sunburned on a cloudy day. For the same reason, it is important to use sunglasses on cloudy days as well as sunny ones, provided there is enough ambient light to see well with sunglasses.

Smoking cigarettes is a strong risk factor for macular degeneration. Some studies have shown that smoking doubles the average risk of developing AMD.[15] The addictive nature of nicotine makes smoking cessation difficult, but a cigarette smoker now has even one more reason to quit: those with early signs of AMD, or with a family history of AMD, can help reduce the risk of central vision blindness by quitting. With over-the-counter and prescription aids, a smoker has assistance available in overcoming the unhealthy habit of smoking.

Vitamin supplements are an excellent way to help protect the eyes from the effects of macular degeneration. While research has provided a good idea of what particular nutrients are the most beneficial for macular degeneration, prior to 2001 no widely conclusive science-based evidence was available. In 2001, the National Eye Institute released the results of a comprehensive study called the Age-Related Eye Disease Study (AREDS). AREDS clearly showed that high levels of antioxidants and zinc significantly reduce the risk of *advanced* age-related macular degeneration. The AREDS formula used in the study included many nutrients already used in existing over-the-counter supplements, but in differing dosages. Today, there are several vitamin manufacturers selling over-the-counter supplements exactly matching the AREDS formula, including Bausch & Lomb PreserVision Vitamins AREDS Formula and Alcon ICaps AREDS Formula. The AREDS formulation includes beta-carotene (25,000 IU), vitamin C (500 mg), vitamin E (400 IU), zinc (80 mg), and cupric oxide (2 mg).

Most eye doctors recommend the use of an AREDS formula vitamin supplement for their macular degeneration patients. Some supplements may increase the chance of lung cancer in smokers, and all users are susceptible to overdosing on vitamin A if multiple supplements are combined. Regular multivitamins do not have high enough dosages of nutrients to take the place of an eye-specific vitamin, nor do eye-specific vitamins have all the nutrients a multivitamin provides for an AMD patient. Typically, it is safe to take both a multivitamin and an AREDS vitamin together, but there are some exceptions, and potential prescription medication interactions exist. Verify the safety of vitamin supplements with your doctor prior to starting supplementation, particularly if you are a smoker.

Lutein, zeaxanthin, and omega-3 fatty acids are additional anti-oxidants believed to be beneficial in macular degeneration, but AREDS did not specifically study these elements. A new, multi-year study is currently under way, which will examine their potential benefits. Many supplements already contain these elements, though their exact benefits are not fully understood.

The original AREDS did not show that vitamin supplements provided any added protection against developing macular degeneration in patients *without* the condition. It only showed benefit to those currently suffering from the disease. Despite this, I still recommend AREDS formulation supplements to my healthy patients who have a family history of AMD but do not currently have signs of AMD themselves. Hopefully, the new study currently underway will shed more light on the role of lutein and other antioxidants in macular degeneration.

Surgery and Medications for Macular Degeneration

Neither the old nor the newer surgical treatments eliminate macular degeneration, but today's surgical and pharmaceutical treatment results are encouraging. Nearly 30–40 percent of patients being treated with injectable drugs for AMD experience some improvement in their visual acuity, and 95 percent are prevented from worsening. No surgical treatments exist for the dry form of AMD. For wet AMD, surgery can act to limit and prevent the leak-prone blood vessel growth in the macular area prior to a bleed occurring. Older surgical treatments involved using a laser to "cauterize" abnormal tissue growth around the macula, thus setting up a barrier and discouraging new blood vessel growth.

A medication called Lucentis (Genentech, Inc.) was approved by the U.S. Food and Drug Administration (FDA) in 2006 for the treatment of "wet" macular degeneration. Lucentis is injected into the eye after local anesthesia and works by blocking the chemical growth factor responsible for the development of new blood vessels in the macula. It hinders the growth of the undesirable blood vessels without doing collateral damage to healthy tissue or to the macula itself. Lucentis is an expensive drug that requires retreatment every four weeks. However, it has actually shown in some cases to allow patients to regain some previously lost visual acuity. An alternate medication named Macugen acts in much the same way, but it is not as effective as Lucentis and is seldom used.

There is some controversy about a third drug that acts very similarly to Lucentis, but is much less expensive. The same company that produces Lucentis also makes a drug called Avastin, which is FDA approved to treat various types of cancer, but is not specifically approved for treating macular degeneration. Though they are not exactly the same drug, they are very similar. Some studies show that Lucentis is slightly more effective than Avastin, but many eye surgeons treat AMD patients "off-label" with Avastin. Avastin's significantly lower cost allows some patients access to this type of treatment that they wouldn't be able to afford with Lucentis.

These newer anti-blood vessel growth treatments have been very effective at limiting the progression of severe macular degeneration. Lucentis and Avastin have undoubtedly preserved eyesight for thousands of people who would have otherwise lost vision more rapidly. Other methods of treating macular degeneration are currently being researched and developed, with many scientists dedicated to discovering a cure. Though dry macular degeneration currently has no prescription or surgical therapies available, treatments are being researched.

Low-Vision Aids

Low vision is a term that broadly defines eyesight that is poor even with the aid of eyeglasses or contact lenses. People who suffer from severely reduced eyesight as a result of macular degeneration are said to have low vision. The two most critical and modifiable factors that help people with low vision to see are increasing magnification and increasing the intensity of light. By optimizing these two factors, they can often function quite well. Hundreds of specialized magnifiers (optical and digital), light sources, and large-print items enable people with AMD to continue functioning independently. Specialized, highly magnified prismatic reading glasses allow the viewing of one letter at a time, and eyeglass-mounted mini-telescopes are often prescribed. Many optometrists specialize in low vision, and perform eye examinations specifically oriented toward low-vision patients. The goal of a low-vision exam is to select and customize the sight-enhancing instruments and products commercially available to help the individual see with their remaining vision. Lifestyle and coping methods to deal with limited eyesight are also detailed. Today's ease of access to computers that allow for adjustable font sizes, and electronic digital readers, such as Amazon.com's Kindle and Apple Computer's iPad, make coping with low vision easier. More information is available online at the Macular Degeneration Partnership (www.amd.org) and at Low Vision Gateway (www.lowvision.org).

PART FOUR

OTHER EYE PROBLEMS

CHAPTER 9

EYE INJURIES
AND FIRST AID

Eye injuries are common, and knowing what to do prior to visiting a doctor will often improve the outcome and recovery period. Contacting an eye doctor or emergency room is the first step to take in all serious eye injuries, with the exception of chemical burns to the eye, which require immediate flushing of the eye with water or saline.

BLUNT TRAUMA TO THE EYE

Blunt injuries to the eye can occur as a result of an automobile accident, a fall, fistfights, sports-related accidents, or any number of other accidents. Fortunately, a strong, bony orbit surrounds and protects the eye, and fat, muscles, and other tissues within the orbit absorb some of the shock from an injury causing compression to the eye. Thus, the eye is well prepared to endure a number of serious injuries.

Black Eye

A "black eye" is the dark discoloration of the skin surrounding the eye as the result of a blunt injury, not an actual blackening of the eye itself. Trauma to the eye, nose, head, or other surrounding tissues are all known to cause black eyes. The loose tissue surrounding the eye swells with fluid and blood, causing the dark and bruised appearance. There is ample space around the eye for leaked blood and fluid to accumulate, which may result in significant swelling and bulging of the eye. The swelling may be severe enough to force the eyelids shut. A black eye may not become apparent immediately after the initial trauma, but may instead develop slowly during the hours afterward. The color of the bruised tissue around the eye will gradually darken from red to deep purple as blood accumulates under the skin and the affected tissues continue to swell. Often the eye appears worse cosmetically than the damage really is; however, it is not wise to merely guess at the extent of an injury, so it is advisable to seek medical attention.

The primary symptoms that accompany a black eye are pain and a feeling of "fullness" around the affected eye, which may last for days. The constant pain and pressure around the eye sometimes cause a headache. Swelling and discoloration normally resolve over the course of several days and weeks after the initial injury.

Serious signs that require an immediate visit to an eye doctor or emergency room include:

- Blurry vision or any reduction of eyesight

- Flashes of light or "floaters" in your vision

- Double vision

- Signs of fluid leaking from the eye

- Inability to move the eye

- Blood visible over the iris, the colored part of the eye (hyphema)

- Significant pain

Cold compresses placed on the eyelids will help reduce the swelling and discomfort by causing the blood vessels to constrict. Use the cold compress for at least fifteen minutes of each hour during the first twenty-four waking hours after the injury. To avoid causing more damage, when placing the cold compresses on the eye wrap ice cubes in a cold washcloth or place a small bag of frozen vegetables in a towel and gently rest it on the affected area.

Penetrating Injuries

Sometimes foreign objects that have penetrated the eye after sustaining an injury are quite obvious, and other times it is impossible to determine by external observation. Objects such as BB pellets or slivers from grinding metal are propelled with great force and can penetrate the eye and come to a rest inside the globe.

If an object such as a piece of metal enters the eye, it is often not found by the doctor until a computerized tomography (CT) scan is performed. In other instances, such as a fishhook lodged in the eye, nothing more than an external examination is needed to detect the foreign object. The doctor will know this, but a magnetic resonance imaging (MRI) scan should not be performed if a metallic foreign body is suspected.

Do not attempt to remove an embedded foreign object yourself, even if it is still partially exposed. Trying to remove a lodged object from the eye without seeking medical attention first will likely be more damaging to an already delicate situation. Attempt to keep the eyes from moving around by looking at a fixed object while someone transports you to medical attention.

FOREIGN BODIES IN THE EYE

From an easily seen eyelash to impossible-to-see fiberglass debris, the types of particles that may accidentally get in the eye are limitless. A foreign object may become lodged in place or move around underneath the eyelids. Metal objects lodged in the cornea commonly form a ring of rust around the area if it is not removed quickly. In many instances of non-embedded foreign bodies, the person may be able to remove the foreign object themselves, or with the help of someone else.

Do's and Don'ts of Removing a Foreign Object from the Eye

- If the individual wears contact lenses, remove the contact lens before attempting to remove the foreign object.

- If the individual has had laser refractive eye surgery (LASIK) in the last year, do not attempt to remove a foreign body without the assistance of a doctor. Depending on the location of the object, it is possible to displace the surgical "flap" that was created during the surgery.

- Try to locate the foreign object by looking in the mirror or asking someone else to look for you.

- Pull the lower eyelid down as the person looks up to determine if the object is underneath the lower lid, then pull the upper eyelid up as the person looks down to inspect beneath the upper lid.

- Instruct the individual to fully look to the left and to the right to inspect the inside and outside corners of the eye.

- Rinse the eye with contact lens or saline solution if available. Make sure the contact lens solution is safe to use directly on the eye. Solutions *not* safe to apply directly to the eye normally have warnings on the bottle. Do not use any eyedrop or solution with a red cap to flush the eye; red-colored caps mean they are not safe to put in the eye (or used only with direct doctor supervision).

- If saline or contact lens solution is not available, flush the eye with distilled or tap water. Have the individual fill their cupped hands with water and lean over a sink to splash water into the eye. A water fountain may be used by holding the upper and lower lids open while leaning over the fountain to flush. If at home, the individual may get in the shower and hold the eye open under a light stream of water to flush the eye.

- If necessary, use the tip of a facial tissue or cotton swab to lightly dab and remove the object. Always swab away from the center of the eye, never toward the center.

- If the object is on the cornea (the clear tissue over the colored iris), do not attempt to remove it. Seek the care of an eye doctor or emergency room medical professional. Attempting to remove a foreign object from the cornea may cause it to become further embedded or scratch the cornea, making removal even more difficult.

- If unable to remove the foreign object yourself, seek medical attention immediately.

- Do not patch the eye, as a patch may hide a developing infection or hemorrhage.

- If the object is removed successfully, monitor for changes in eyesight or lingering redness, pain, or discharge from the eye. If the foreign object was accompanied by an abrasion of ocular tissue, an infection may occur even after the object is removed. Seek medical attention if there is excessive light sensitivity, pain, or discharge from the eye.

CORNEAL ABRASIONS

The cornea is the clear tissue that covers the colored iris. Millions of pain-receptor nerves are located in this tissue, the purpose of which is to cause immediate awareness of any threat to the well-being of the corneal tissue. Even the smallest corneal abrasions are extremely painful and have the capacity to debilitate the toughest of men. Fortunately, the cornea has the wonderful ability to heal itself swiftly. Most abrasions do not cause permanent scarring or long-term vision loss when they are treated properly and promptly. However, severe injuries to the cornea may leave scarring that permanently damages or destroys eyesight.

Treatment of a corneal abrasion involves removing any remaining foreign objects in the eye, preventing infections with antibiotics, managing pain, and facilitating the healing process. Constant eyelid movement over the abrasion slows the healing process and further agitates the wound. Often, the doctor will place a "bandage" contact lens on the eye for overnight wear to create a shield over the abrasion. This hastens the healing process and helps alleviate pain. In addition, doctors may dilate the affected eye with a long-lasting dilation eyedrop to aid in pain reduction. Over-the-counter or prescription oral pain medications are normally recommended to control significant pain.

Corneal abrasions are best managed by a doctor rather than by self-treatment. Given the potential chance for a secondary infection as well as the possibility of long-term scarring, it is advisable to be safe and have it evaluated by an eye-care provider.

SUBCONJUNCTIVAL HEMORRHAGE

Subconjunctival hemorrhages are common occurrences and are often startling to the individual when first detected. A subconjunctival hemorrhage is commonly referred to as a "burst blood vessel" on the sclera (the white part of the eye). Though the sclera is mostly colorless, there are small and large blood vessels that run

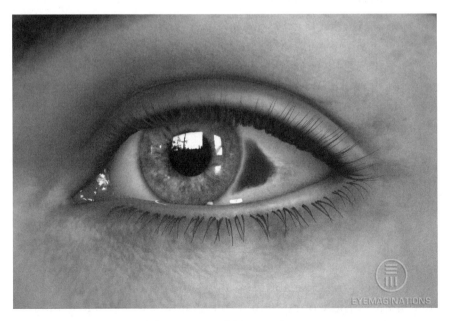

Subconjunctival Hemmorhage

through and above the tissue. Much like a bruise, a subconjuncti-val hemorrhage is blood spilled out of one of these vessels, which subsequently accumulates under the transparent conjunctiva (the thin, clear tissue layer covering the white sclera). Blood is trapped between these two tissues and the bright red appearance and dis-persion of blood is disturbing upon observation.

Subconjunctival hemorrhages are usually painless, but a feel-ing of fullness or pressure on the eye is frequently reported as a result of the extra blood volume between the sclera and con-junctiva. The vision is rarely affected, but the deep red appearance of the eye usually generates comments from others. Fortunately, subconjunctival hemorrhages are self-limiting and typically only require monitoring.

A hemorrhage of this nature may take two to three weeks to resolve, similar to a bruise elsewhere on the body. A skin bruise looks "black and blue" because of the overlying fat, muscle, and skin, but a subconjunctival hemorrhage allows an unobstructed view of the blood. During the initial hours and days after the blood vessel rupture, the redness may slowly spread out to encompass larger areas of the whites of the eye, giving the appearance of it worsening. Over the course of a few weeks, the body naturally resorbs the blood, and it is common for the hemorrhage to change in color and brightness during the healing process.

There are various causes for a subconjunctival hemorrhage, and it is frequently difficult to pinpoint the exact cause. Most epi-sodes are random occurrences that may be traced back to a Valsava maneuver. A Valsalva maneuver is any attempt to exhale while keeping the airway closed. Lifting a heavy object, vomiting, heavy coughing, heavy sneezing, or straining during a bowel movement are all known causes of a subconjunctival hemorrhage. A Valsalva maneuver temporarily increases the pressure in the veins, subse-quently causing a blood vessel in the eye to rupture. Ocular trauma or eye surgery may also cause subconjunctival hemorrhages.

People who bruise easily are predisposed to subconjunctival hemorrhages, and individuals taking blood thinners are particularly susceptible. Users of blood thinners, anticoagulants, or aspirin may have a difficult time getting the ruptured blood vessel in the eye to stop bleeding and should notify their eye-care provider and physician, who will determine whether it is safe to temporarily stop taking those medications until the hemorrhage stops bleeding.

Permanent ocular damage rarely results from a subconjunctival hemorrhage. However, multiple episodes may indicate underlying problems such as high blood pressure or blood disorders and should be evaluated by a doctor. See your eye-care provider if you have a history of high blood pressure or if you experience:

- Decreased vision with the hemorrhage

- Blood leaking out of your eye (subconjunctival hemorrhages don't cause blood to leak out of the eye)

- Multiple episodes of subconjunctival hemorrhages

- Ocular pain

- A subconjunctival hemorrhage simultaneously in both eyes

BURNS

Chemical Burns of the Eye

Approximately 10 percent of eye injuries are caused by burns to the eye, often from chemical substances. Many common household and workplace chemicals cause significant damage, including blindness, upon contact with the eye. Prompt medical attention is necessary to achieve the best recovery from a chemical burn.

Chemicals have a pH rating that ranges between 0 and 14; 7.0 is considered a "neutral" pH. Acidic solutions have a pH of less than 7.0, and alkaline (basic) solutions have a pH higher than 7.0. While neither acidic nor alkaline burns are good, alkaline burns are the most damaging to the ocular tissues. Alkaline burns of the eyelid and ocular tissue can continue to cause tissue damage even after the initial chemical has been flushed from the tissue.

Alkaline substances include:

- Lye (oven cleaners, liquid drain cleaners)
- Ammonia (household window and cleaning solutions)
- Lime (fertilizers)

Acidic substances include:

- Car battery acid
- Nail polish remover
- Vinegar

The initial treatment for alkaline and acid burns of the eye is the same: *immediately flush the affected eyes with saline solution or water for at least ten minutes and then seek medical care.* As long as the chemical is present, it will continue to do damage to ocular tissues, so *removing the damaging substance as quickly as possible is of the utmost importance to minimize the risk of permanent damage to the eye.*

Use the most sterile solution readily available to flush the eye:

- Saline solution or contact lens storage solution
- An eyewash station (lean over a water fountain if an eyewash station is not available)
- An eyewash bottle in a first aid kit

If a shower is available, enter the shower (with clothes on) and stand under the showerhead set a with low-pressure stream.

Hold the eye(s) open to allow proper flushing for at least ten minutes. Have another person transport you to emergency medical care or call an ambulance while the eye is being flushed.

Try to determine what type of substance got in the eye and proceed to the closest emergency room. The doctor's treatment plan is determined by the agent that burned the eye. Medical treatment

includes continued flushing of the eyes until the pH of the eyes
returns to normal. The doctor will attempt to obtain a visual acuity measurement and examine the affected tissues. A measurement
of the intraocular pressure may be obtained. Often, the eye is
dilated with prescription drops for a day or more to help control
pain. Antibiotic drops or ointment are used to prevent an infection
of the compromised tissue, and ocular steroids may be used to
quiet inflammation and facilitate healing. Oral pain medications
are often required for several days, depending on the severity of
the burn.

Thermal (Heat) Burns of the Eye

Heat burns the eye in the same way that heat and fire can singe our
skin. It's painful *just to think* about a burn of the eye! Thermal
burns of the ocular tissues may be caused by:

- Flames

- Explosions, including fireworks

- Steam/hot air

- Curling irons

- Cigarettes

Thermal burns often affect the skin of the eyelid as much or
more than the eye itself. Flushing the eye with water is important
if foreign bodies, such as particles from fireworks or ashes, are suspected in the eye. Otherwise, heat burns from steam or a curling
iron do not require flushing. A cold compress will soothe the pain
of the eye and affected eyelids during transportation to medical
care. As with burns of the skin, any thermal burn of the cornea,
conjunctiva, or eyelids should be examined by an eye-care pro -
vider or emergency room physician. Proper medical management
will help reduce the pain and potential for long-term scarring or
tissue damage.

Eye Protection

No discussion about ocular injuries and burns would be complete without some mention of eye protection and safety. The overwhelming majority of burns and injuries to the eyes are avoidable with proper eye protection. While we can never be fully prepared for the host of accidents that may occur, it is wise to take precautions when increased risks are known. Using eye protection when handling car batteries and household cleaning agents can save your eyes from pain, damage, and even blindness.

Irritants and Ocular Burns

The cornea has an amazing ability to regenerate new tissue and recover from various types of trauma. Irritants such as pepper spray and smoke may cause considerable discomfort to the eyes, but they rarely cause long-term harm. Many corneal burns heal well and leave no permanent damage either. However, permanent damage or even blindness may occur in severe chemical or thermal burns of the eye. Severe burns may require a corneal transplant to restore eyesight to a heavily scarred eye. When in doubt about seeking medical care for mild to moderate burns, err on the side of caution and see a doctor.

RECURRENT CORNEAL EROSIONS

A recurrent corneal erosion (RCE) occurs when the eye causes a corneal abrasion to itself. It is very similar to a corneal abrasion, with the exception that the RCE abrasion comes from inside the eye rather than from outside. This "self-scratching" of the cornea can happen in recurring episodes with varying intervals of every few days to every few years.

The symptoms of a corneal erosion usually include a recurring history of an acute, stabbing pain upon opening the eyes when waking from sleep. Excessive tearing, blurred vision, and light sensitivity usually accompany the eye pain. The pain often subsides as the day proceeds with the eyes frequently feeling "back to normal" prior to the end of the day.

Recurrent corneal erosions are often difficult to diagnose initially since they appear the same to a doctor as an externally caused corneal abrasion. If the eye is not examined soon after the initial acute pain, the cornea heals so rapidly that the abrasion may become invisible to the doctor by later in the day.

The tissue of the cornea is approximately the thickness of a fingernail. It is made up of five layers, the outermost being the epithelium. The cells in the cornea are stacked tightly and are held together by molecular elements, similar to bricks and mortar. Normally, the connections between the cells in the cornea are air-tight, but under abnormal circumstances the cells form gaps between them like cracked mortar in a brick wall. These cellular "cracks" allow microscopic water droplets to form in the cornea. As the microscopic droplets develop, they eventually rise to the surface of the cornea, where they rupture and release their contents. The rupturing droplets cause breaks in the epithelium and scratch the eye's surface. At the moment these micro-erosions occur, the eye becomes intensely painful, light sensitive, and red, just as in an externally caused corneal abrasion.

Recurrent corneal erosions are caused by disruption in the cellular arrangement of the cornea. The disruption is due to an abnormal functioning or cellular formation called a corneal dystrophy, or as the result of previous corneal trauma. Most individuals suffering from a recurrent corneal erosion are able to pinpoint their first painful episode as being subsequent to an eye injury or external corneal abrasion.

Treatment of RCEs is tailored to the severity and frequency of episodes. The pain of the erosion is treated the same way as an abrasion caused by external sources. Normal treatment protocol includes dilating the eye, prescribing topical or oral pain medications and antibiotics, and the use of a "bandage" contact lens.

Long-term treatments may include using eyedrops containing a high level of salt to help draw excess fluid out of the cornea prior to an eruption forming. Another alternative treatment is anterior stromal puncture, a procedure that causes the cells in the cornea to reorganize. Stromal puncture can significantly reduce painful erosion episodes for many individuals.

FLOATERS

Floaters are another name for small, black, cobweb-like disturbances that appear to be darting around in the eyesight. They may abruptly appear seemingly out of nowhere, but then refuse to go away once they have arrived.

The fluid in back of the eye is called the vitreous humor. This thick, clear, jelly-like fluid sometimes develops pockets of water and other disturbances that cause visual distortions. These floaters in the vitreous fluid move around in the eye much like fake snow particles in a winter snow globe, though fewer in number. In the absence of flashes of light or a more significant visual impairment, floaters are often more of a nuisance than a serious health concern. They can significantly improve as time passes, and many people are less bothered as they become adjusted to them. Vitreous floaters commonly break up into smaller particles over months and years, which helps make them less noticeable as well. However, some larger floaters never seem to subside and individuals continue to be bothered by them over time.

POSTERIOR VITREOUS DETACHMENT

A posterior vitreous detachment may also cause floaters. The vitreous fluid in the eye is firmly attached at a specific area at the back of the eye (the optic nerve). The vitreous is also firmly attached in a 360-degree band toward the front of the inside of the eye. In all other areas inside the eye, the vitreous fluid is loosely attached.

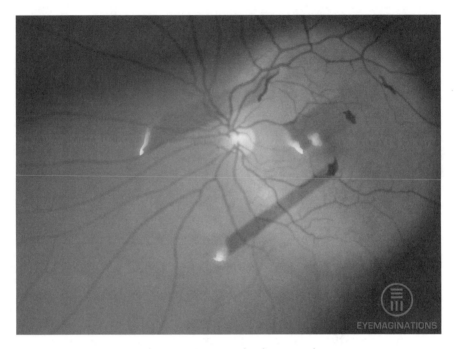

Vitreous Floaters Casting Shadows on the Retina

Risk factors for posterior vitreous detachment include:

- Age progression, particularly over age fifty

- High levels of myopia (–6.00 diopters and higher), but any level of myopia is a risk

- Eye or head injuries, particularly jarring injuries such as being involved in an auto accident

- Eye surgery, particularly cataract surgery

A posterior vitreous detachment occurs when the vitreous fluid "breaks loose" of its firm attachment at the optic nerve. The traction on the retina caused by the vitreous fluid pulling away from it may cause the perception of flashes of light. Any perception of flashing lights should be examined immediately, since it may be an indication of a more serious retinal problem.

When the vitreous detaches from the retina at the optic nerve, a wrinkle-like distortion occurs in the area of the vitreous fluid where it was once attached. The wrinkle scatters light entering the eye and casts a shadow on the retina, which is perceived as the floater. Floaters are shadows of the debris in the eye.

The doctor's diagnosis of a posterior vitreous detachment involves a thorough medical history and description of the appearance of the floaters or flashes of light in the eye. Through a dilated pupil, the eye doctor will examine the vitreous fluid and retina using a combination of lenses along with a microscope and a head loupe separately. In most cases of floaters caused by a posterior vitreous detachment, the doctor will be able to observe the floaters during the examination, although sometimes the floaters "hide" because the vitreous fluid moves around.

Upon initial suspicion, vitreous detachments require proper

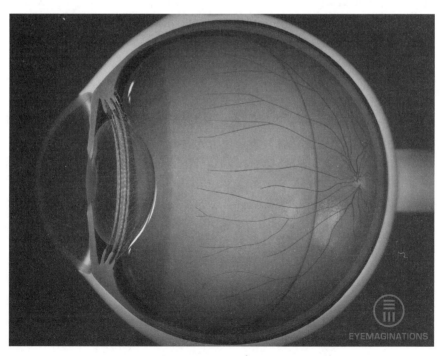

Vitreous Detachment

diagnosis by an eye doctor to rule out more serious retinal damage. The eye doctor will also be able to inspect the eye for any retinal tears or damage that may have occurred along with the onset of floaters. Further medical intervention is usually not required for floaters alone. Extremely debilitating floaters may warrant surgical intervention, but this is uncommon. The risks of surgery for floaters far outweigh the potential benefits for all but the smallest percentage of the population.

RETINAL DETACHMENTS

Many people have heard of a retinal detachment and are familiar enough with the term to know that it is a serious condition. Retinal detachments can potentially cause blindness, but modern technical advancements allow eye surgeons to repair detachments and restore eyesight to many people. A retinal detachment is a medical emergency and must be managed immediately. Approximately one out of every 15,000 people in the United States suffers from a retinal detachment.

The retina is the thin layer lining the inside of the eye that perceives light. Similar to the film in a 35 mm camera, the function of the retina is to receive the image focused on it from the lenses at the front of the eye. The retina then transports the visual information to the brain via the optic nerve. The retina is attached to underlying layers of tissue inside the eye. However, trauma or stretching of the retina may cause it to detach from the underlying layers.

Symptoms of a Retinal Detachment

Unless it is precipitated by trauma, a retinal detachment does not cause pain. The detachment may happen spontaneously, particularly in individuals with high levels of myopia. Individuals with a retinal detachment describe seeing lightning-bolt or arc-like flashes of white light in their peripheral vision. A severe retinal detachment will also make the eyesight go "black" in the field of view that corresponds to the detached area of retina. If a significant area of retina is detached, the individual may describe their eyesight looking like a curtain or a veil obscuring a large part of their vision. Most retinal detachments occur in the peripheral retina, causing the shadows and flashes of light to appear in the peripheral parts of the vision. The detached areas of retina no longer transmit visual information to the brain, causing blindness in those areas. Rare detachments of the entire retina cause total blindness.

Diagnosis of a retinal detachment occurs with a doctor's careful examination of the retina through a dilated pupil. The patient's symptoms of flashes of light or obscured vision will alert the doctor to specifically examine the retina for a tear or detachment. The doctor may take photographs of the retina and perform a computerized visual field examination to aid in the diagnosis.

Risk factors for retinal detachments include:

- Significant myopia (–6.00 diopters or higher)

- Aging—most common over age forty

- Trauma—recent or past trauma to the eye or head

- Previous eye surgery, such as cataract surgery or refractive surgery

- A history of retinal detachment in one eye (increases the odds of a subsequent detachment in the other eye)

- A diagnosis of degenerative peripheral retinal tissue, such as lattice degeneration or retinoschisis

- Ocular tumors or metastasis

- Family history of retinal detachments

Trauma is a well-known cause of retinal detachments. Injuries to the head or eye may jar the head so profoundly that the retina detaches. Boxers who repeatedly get hit in the head are at high risk of suffering from retinal detachments. Though the retina does not transmit pain, the injury certainly will. A traumatic retinal detachment causes the same type of symptoms that a spontaneous retinal detachment does.

Treatment of Retinal Detachments

Rapid detection aids in the prognosis for recovery from a retinal detachment. A retinal specialist will surgically reattach the retina to the inside of the eye. The reattachment of the retina may be accomplished by several different means, depending on the location and severity of the detachment:

- Thermal laser applied to the inside of the eye, which "tacks" the retina back in place.

- Cryopexy uses a cold probe (rather than the heat of a laser) to "tack" the retina back in place. Cryopexy is applied from the exterior of the eye.

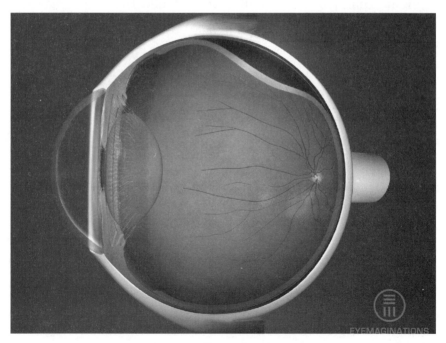

Retinal Detachment

- Pneumatic retinopexy involves inserting a gas bubble into the eye that holds the retina in place until reattachment occurs via the body's own healing process. Over time, the gas bubble dissipates while the retina remains intact. This method involves extremely limited head movement for up to several weeks at a time, to insure that the gas bubble does not move around in the eye.

- Scleral buckling is a surgical technique that involves inserting a medical-grade band around the eye to bring the retina and internal tissues back into position. The scleral buckle remains intact indefinitely.

Patients with known risk factors for retinal detachment should have annual dilated eye examinations to monitor for changes or increasing risk factors for retinal detachment. At the doctor's recommendation, some people may require dilated examinations more than once a year. Patients at high risk for retinal detachment are selectively treated with prophylactic retinal laser surgery to minimize the risks of developing an impending detachment.

LONG-TERM EFFECTS OF OCULAR INJURIES

Long-term ocular health concerns may develop years after sustaining an ocular injury. Blunt trauma injuries to the eye and face may increase the risk of cataracts and glaucoma several months or years after the injury. Individuals who have sustained head injuries from fistfights, sports-related injuries, automobile accidents, or other accidents need to be especially vigilant about having annual vision and ocular health examinations to monitor for these conditions.

Traumatic Cataracts

Long after a contusion of the eye or head has healed, a gradual haziness of vision may develop, possibly indicating cataract formation subsequent to the injury. The tissue of the physiological lens inside the eye is sensitive to disruption or manipulation of any kind. As in eye injuries, various types of eye surgery sometimes increase the odds of developing a cataract simply because the lens is so sensitive. Electrocution is a well-known cause of cataract formation, as well. The management and treatment of a traumatic cataract is no different than for cataracts caused by other means.

Traumatic Glaucoma

In addition to cataracts, contusions of the eye are also associated with a higher lifetime risk of developing glaucoma. Injuries to the eye may damage the eye's internal drainage mechanism, which in turn causes the intraocular pressure to elevate. Depending on the severity and nature of the ocular injury, glaucoma may develop immediately after the injury. In other cases, glaucoma may take months or years to cause the intraocular pressure to increase. Be sure to relate any history of severe head or ocular trauma to the eye doctor.

Recurrent Corneal Erosions Caused by Previous Eye Injury

Once the pain and visual disturbances of a corneal abrasion have healed, a disruption of the corneal cells may still remain indefinitely. Microscopic pockets of fluid sometimes develop within the abnormal corneal tissue, subsequently leading to episodes of extreme pain in the eye that may last for hours or days. Short- and long-term treatments exist (see "Recurrent Corneal Erosions" on page 179).

CHAPTER 10

INFECTIONS

CONJUNCTIVITIS

The conjunctiva is a clear, thin mucous membrane that covers the whites of the eyes and the underside of the eyelids. This tissue is susceptible to infection by bacteria and viruses just as our sinuses, ears, and throats may be infected. Commonly referred to as "pink-eye," conjunctivitis comes in many forms and from many causes, including bacteria, viruses, and allergies. (Conjunctivitis was also covered in Chapter 6. See that chapter for more information on allergic conjunctivitis.) Eye irritants such as pool chlorine, smoke, shampoo, and soaps may also cause conjunctivitis.

Newborns may develop bacterial conjunctivitis as they pass through the birth canal if the mother has gonorrhea or chlamydia. These sexually transmitted diseases are bacterial in nature and often the mother is treated during pregnancy prior to giving birth, preventing transmission to the newborn. However, a mother's sexually transmitted disease diagnosis is not always made prior to giving birth. For this reason, antibiotic ointment is administered to infants' eyes just after birth to prophylactically treat any bacteria that may have passed to the newborn.

In all types of conjunctivitis, the eyes are uncomfortable and the whites of the eyes are red, giving anywhere from a light pink up to a bright red appearance (hence, the name "pink-eye"). Symptoms of conjunctivitis may include frequent tearing, pain, light sensitivity, discharge, swelling and/or matting shut of the eyelids, and itching.

Bacterial Conjunctivitis

Conjunctivitis in children is usually caused by bacteria. The bacteria that cause eye infections are often the same ones that cause sinus, throat, and ear infections. Bacterial conjunctivitis can develop quickly and may cause significant crusting of the eyelids, yellow to green discharge of pus during the day, and matting shut of the eyelids at night so that they are difficult to open upon waking in the morning. Bacterial conjunctivitis is contagious and is easily spread to the unaffected eye and to other people. I advise patients with bacterial (and viral) conjunctivitis to behave the same way they would when they have a cold: wash your hands frequently, don't shake hands with others, and don't share towels, washcloths, and pillowcases with others. Also, don't rub or wipe the infected eye and then rub the unaffected eye, as it will become cross-infected.

Parents should consider keeping children home from school for forty-eight hours after starting antibiotic eyedrops to prevent the infection from spreading to other people. Conjunctivitis spreads quickly through schools and daycare centers, but the spread of pink-eye is mitigated if the child stays home for a couple of days.

Bacterial conjunctivitis will likely go away on its own within two weeks, but treatment with prescription antibiotic eyedrops clears the infection in half the time or less and reduces the exposure of others to the contagious infection. Visiting your child's eye-care provider or pediatrician at the first sign of an eye infection is strongly recommended.

Viral Conjunctivitis

Viral conjunctivitis has many of the same symptoms as bacterial conjunctivitis, but whereas viral eye infections make the eyes look pink in color, bacterial infections make the eyes more red than pink. Another difference between viral and bacterial infections is that viral infections cause more excessive tearing, with little to no pus. Bacterial infections usually involve heavy amounts of pus.

Viral eye infections may last anywhere from a few days up to several months. Like all viruses, there are not many treatment options for this type of infection other than cold compresses to soothe the eyes. Infrequently, a doctor may use steroid eye drops in an attempt to make a very uncomfortable eye feel better, but it does not alter the course of the virus. A newer treatment option that is "off-label"—not specifically approved by the U.S. Food and Drug Administration (FDA)—and has reportedly excellent results is using a diluted solution of Betadine, which is directly applied to the eye as an eyedrop in the doctor's office. Betadine is an iodine solution that is widely used as a sterilization preparation on the skin prior to a surgical procedure.

STYE

The medical name for a stye is "hordeolum." Each of the four eyelids has approximately twenty glands that secrete oil through ducts exiting just behind our eyelashes. The glands' oil mixes with our tears to form a healthy tear barrier. The oil prevents the watery part of our tears from evaporating off of our eyes, thus retaining the moisture. A stye occurs when one of the oil glands gets blocked and subsequently becomes infected.

Styes typically begin by forming a small knot or bump on the eyelid around the area of infection. Over several days, redness and tenderness develop as the stye becomes more pronounced in size and fills with infected material. Initially, styes are painful only when touched or manipulated, but as they grow in size the pain may become constant. Though the eyelid is infected, this condition is not usually contagious unless discharge from the stye comes in contact with healthy tissue.

The two classifications of styes are external and internal. External styes typically form a "whitehead" at the margin of the eyelid

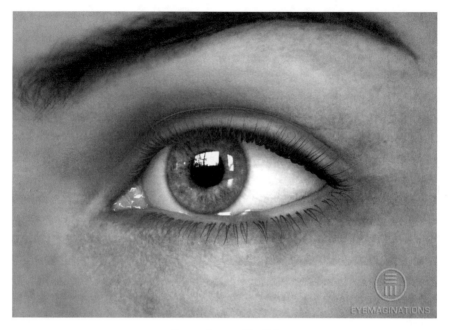

Stye—Lower Eyelid

much the same way a pimple does on the skin. Internal styes are deeper infections of the gland that do not extend all the way to its orifice. External styes are usually easier to treat at home than internal styes, since draining the stye can often cause the infection to resolve.

The same initial methods are used to treat both external and internal styes. Hot compresses are used in an attempt to cause the stye to form a "whitehead" so that the infected material can be drained from the gland. With gentle pressure from a cotton swab (just after applying a hot compress), the gland may be coerced to express the infected material. This relieves the pressure and pain associated with the stye and often allows the body to heal the remaining inflammation. However, if the infection is widespread and some infectious material remains in the gland after drainage, the gland will continue to produce more pus and will not likely heal without prescription antibiotics. If hot compresses are unsuccessful at resolving the infection after several days, it is important to be treated by a doctor. Since the infection of a stye is internal to the eyelid, antibiotic eyedrops and ointments are rarely effective methods at treating the infection. Instead, oral antibiotics will likely be prescribed by the doctor.

It is important to address and treat a stye promptly. Mild styes can fester for several weeks without growing much larger, but if that is allowed to occur the stye can metamorphose into a chalazion.

Chalazion

A chalazion is a "matured" stye. Most styes resolve after a one or two weeks. Some styes require prescription antibiotics, but milder may not. If the stye remains for weeks or months, the pus trapped inside the gland turns into granular material that the body usually can't remove on its own. The acute infection from the stye may clear, but the remaining internal material caused by the infection can remain indefinitely. Chalazia produce a knot on the eyelid

Hot Compress Instructions

Saturate a washcloth with the warmest tap water tolerable without causing a burn to the skin. Eyelid skin is very thin, so err on the side of cooler rather than hotter if you are unsure of the temperature initially. Wring out the washcloth and fold it in quarters. Close your eyes and rest the hot washcloth on the affected area of the eyelid for approximately ten minutes. You may need to refold the washcloth several times to keep the hottest part of it applied to the eyelid. Do not hesitate to run the washcloth under hot water multiple times as it cools. The hot compresses should be applied at least four times a day, but more if your schedule allows. A tip some people use is hard-boiling an egg, and then wrapping the egg in a warm washcloth before applying it to the eyelid. The egg will retain the heat for an extended period of time so you won't have to constantly rewet and refold the washcloth.

similar to a stye, but they are painless to the touch and are often not as red in color. Once the acutely painful stye has turned to a painless chalazion, more drastic measures usually have to be taken to remove it.

As with styes, the first line of treatment of a chalazion is hot compresses for several days, if that has not previously been attempted. They rarely respond well to hot compresses, but they occasionally improve. Chalazia do not respond to topical or oral antibiotics since the infection has already cleared and only the material byproducts of the previous infection remain. If the hot compresses don't eliminate the knot, then a surgeon will either reduce the chalazion with an injection of steroids or surgically lance it to remove the internal contents.

BLEPHARITIS

Blepharitis is also an infection of the eyelids, but it affects the skin rather than the internal eyelid glands. Blepharitis is a relatively common condition that occurs when the normal bacterial counts on the skin become overgrown. Under healthy conditions, our skin maintains a baseline level of bacteria, mostly staphylococcus. Warm, moist environments allow bacteria to flourish, and the eyelids provide the ideal setting for the bacteria to thrive above normal levels.

Blepharitis is both inflammatory and infectious, though not contagious in nature. Symptoms of blepharitis may include redness and swelling of the eyelids, as well as flakiness of eyelid skin at the edges of the lids near the eyelashes. The eyelid inflammation from blepharitis also causes irritation, itchiness, and general discomfort in varying degrees. The lids characteristically appear to have a pinkish-red hue to them as if they've just been rubbed vigorously. Though chronic in nature, blepharitis "comes and goes" with intermittent periods ranging from normalcy up through rampant inflammation. A flare-up of blepharitis may last for several weeks and then subside, only to return a short time later. Though the level of inflammation fluctuates, it can be difficult to eliminate all recurrences even with prescription medications.

Blepharitis is found most commonly in people who work in dusty environments, those with oily skin, people with acne rosacea, or those with poor hygiene. Often, none of those conditions are present, yet blepharitis still exists. There are several types and classifications of blepharitis, but the symptoms and treatment are all relatively similar.

The severity of eyelid inflammation dictates the level of treatment required to manage both the acute and chronic symptoms of blepharitis. The mainstay of blepharitis management is the frequent use of lid scrubs with non-irritating shampoo. Hot compresses and lid scrubs help remove the excess bacteria, oil, and flaking skin that are prevalent in blepharitis.

Lid scrubs are available in commercially prepared premoistened pads or foams found at pharmacies and grocery stores (Ocusoft makes several commercially available products). A less expensive, but less convenient, method is to lather baby shampoo on a warm washcloth and gently scrub the eyelids. Initially, the lid scrubs should be repeated 3–4 times per day until improvement is noted. As the inflammation is controlled, less frequent lid scrubs may keep the inflammation under control. If the lid scrubs alone are insufficient to control the blepharitis, an eye doctor may prescribe oral antibiotic medications or antibiotic and steroid ophthalmic ointment to treat the eyelids.

Like dandruff, flakes of dry skin often become trapped in the base of the eyelashes of individuals with blepharitis. The dandruff-like flakes further trap bacteria that aggravate the condition. Frequent lid scrubs will remove the bacteria, oil, and skin flakes to help control the inflammation. In addition to the lid scrubs, a cotton swab moistened with warm water is also helpful in removing the flakes from the base of the eyelashes.

Many eye doctors recommend taking omega-3 essential fatty acid supplements in an attempt to help control chronic blepharitis. Omega-3 supplements are known to help aid in the proper function and regulation of the eyelid glands. Many people have alleviated symptoms of blepharitis and dry eyes by increasing their intake of omega-3s. Certain types of blepharitis are known to be caused by a dysfunction of the eyelid glands, so it is common to suffer from both dry eyes and blepharitis simultaneously. The eye-care provider often needs to manage both conditions, and fortunately lid scrubs and omega-3 supplementation seem to help each of these conditions.

KERATITIS

Keratitis is inflammation or irritation of the cornea. Keratitis may be classified as infectious (caused by an offending organism) or "sterile." Sterile keratitis is inflammation due to non-organic causes such as lack of oxygen, ultraviolet (UV) light exposure, or abrasions. This discussion concentrates on infectious keratitis.

Just as the skin functions as the body's natural barrier and defense against infection, the cornea is the eye's barrier. And, like a cut in the skin causes a breach in the body's defenses, the clear cornea is susceptible to being infringed upon by various organisms, including bacteria, viruses, and even fungi. Though infections by these organisms can usually be treated, corneal scarring may be left in the wake of an infection. Depending on the location and size of the corneal scar, permanent impairment or blindness may result.

Viral Keratitis

Viral keratitis is commonly caused by the herpes simplex or herpes zoster virus. Once a person is infected with a herpes virus, it continues to exist in the body indefinitely, though often in a dormant state. Stress and other causes may reactivate the herpes virus. Herpes simplex is the most common type of viral keratitis; this virus is also well known for causing cold sores around the mouth. If the simplex virus becomes activated in the eye, the cornea is attacked and is slowly eaten away by the virus, causing ulceration of the cornea. Herpes simplex virus (HSV) keratitis is extremely painful and often affects vision. In addition to eye pain, common symptoms include tearing, light sensitivity, redness, and swelling of the affected eye. Rapid diagnosis and treatment are critical since the potential for long-term scarring is high if the infection is not brought under control in a timely manner.

Most viruses that attack the body do not respond well to medication and are left to "run their course." Fortunately, though, effective treatments, including both eyedrop and oral antiviral medications, help manage this type of ocular viral infection. It is clinically challenging to bring a severe case of HSV keratitis under control, making early diagnosis vital. Some individuals have only one episode of HSV keratitis that never returns, but for many the keratitis will reappear. Each subsequent episode of keratitis increases the odds of another future recurrence. After the initial episode, the individual should be on alert to the early symptoms of a recurrence and seek medical care immediately.

Bacterial Keratitis

Bacterial keratitis occurs when the corneal surface is breached, allowing bacteria to infect the underlying corneal tissue. Ulceration occurs when the bacteria carves out the corneal tissue. Some bacteria, such as *Pseudomonas,* are so aggressive that they are capable of "eating" their way entirely through the cornea, causing perforation. Improper care, handling, or disinfection of contact lenses are frequently cited as underlying causes of bacterial keratitis. Stretching the replacement schedule of contact lenses beyond the doctor's prescribed interval is a well-known factor in the incidence as well. Today's highly effective antibiotics are able to control most cases of bacterial keratitis, but aggressive bacterial ulcers are still capable of causing blindness even with proper treatment.

Acanthamoeba Keratitis

Acanthamoeba is a protozoa that is known to aggressively attack the corneal tissue. Infections are particularly dangerous, sometimes requiring hospitalization. *Acanthamoeba* infections are also usually associated with improper contact lens use and disinfection. Since *Acanthamoeba* is found in fresh water, infections are sometimes linked to using a hot tub or swimming in pools or natural bodies of water while wearing contact lenses.

While often difficult to treat, a "cocktail" of multiple topical antibiotics can sometimes overcome an ocular *Acanthamoeba* infection. Many individuals with *Acanthamoeba* infections of the cornea have such significant scarring that a corneal transplant is required to restore normal eyesight.

Fungal Keratitis

Fungal keratitis is very rare but may be caused when vegetative material, such as a tree branch or pine needle, scratches the cornea.

In 2006, Renu MoistureLoc contact lens solution was recalled from store shelves because it was thought to be associated with a rare outbreak of fungal keratitis across the United States. Over 150 cases of fungal keratitis were diagnosed, though investigators from the U.S. Centers for Disease Control and Prevention (CDC) concluded that the Renu MoistureLoc formulation had not been contaminated. Though still uncertain, it is suspected that poor patient compliance combined with the use of Renu MoistureLoc solutions were causative factors.

Though the condition is difficult to manage, antifungal eye-drops can help rein in fungal keratitis.

CHAPTER 11

YOUR EYES
AND HEADACHES

Headaches vary widely in their symptoms and location, and because the causes of headaches are so numerous, a list of causative factors would be practically endless. Since the eye is a direct neurological extension of the brain, it makes sense that the eyes and brain are often interconnected with reference to headaches. It goes both ways—eye problems can cause headaches, and headaches can cause eye problems.

EYE PROBLEMS CAUSING HEADACHES

A common symptom that prompts people to seek an eye examination is a recent onset of headaches. Most headaches that are caused by the eyes produce pain in the forehead area. It is rare for the eyes to be the source of the headache if it primarily affects the sides, top, or back of the head.

The most frequently observed ocular cause of headaches is a change of vision prescription that has not yet been corrected for. All types of vision prescription shifts are capable of causing frequent headaches. An outdated vision prescription for contact lenses or eyeglasses that is too weak or too strong is usually the cause. When the vision correction is too weak, we often reflexively and unconsciously squint to make the slightly blurry images clear. Squinting causes a constant tightening of the facial and ocular muscles, which can subsequently lead to a headache. Alternatively, a vision prescription that is too strong causes the internal muscles of the eyes to contract, forcing them to work much harder in an attempt to overcome the additional prescription. Many people have temporarily tried on someone else's glasses and instantly experienced the "headachy" discomfort that results from overcorrection.

Uncorrected or improperly corrected astigmatism can also be blamed for headaches. Astigmatism causes images to have multiple focal points in the same eye. This is a difficult challenge for the eye to resolve without a vision-correcting lens and is well known to be a source of chronic headaches until it is fixed.

Around age forty, individuals whose eyes are beginning to lose the natural ability to focus near images (a condition known as presbyopia) will often describe headaches as the earliest symptom. As presbyopia develops, the internal eye muscles struggle to bring close images into focus, but the effort required exceeds the eye's ability and headaches may result.

Binocularity problems of the visual system are another potential ocular source of headaches. Binocularity issues typically cause pain around the eyes and forehead area. Our ability to receive a separate image from each of the eyes, and then fuse them into one "stereo" image, is an amazing neurological feat. It is a complex method whereby the neurological and muscular systems of our eyes and brain must work in perfect concert. When this complex process is dysfunctional, overwhelming stress is placed on the visual system. As a prerequisite to binocular vision, the six eye muscles attached to each eye must work in perfect conjunction with the six muscles of the other eye. The ocular muscles are not always capable of providing the proper amount of eye positioning necessary in a binocular disorder, and the additional ocular stress may lead to headaches. One of the most commonly diagnosed binocular problems leading to headaches while reading is called convergence insufficiency (see Chapter 6 for more information).

During a vision and ocular health examination, most eye

doctors ask patients if they suffer from headaches. The more detail the doctor receives regarding the headaches, the easier it is to differentiate the ocular diagnosis related to the headache, if they are connected. Patients who complain of headaches often receive additional testing that may not otherwise be performed during a comprehensive eye examination.

Though most eye-related headaches are located at the front of the head, headaches emanating from the neck or back of the head may also be related to the eyes, at least indirectly. Reading or working on a computer for long hours requires us to sit in exactly the same position for extended periods to keep our eyes focused on the reading material. If the body's posture is incorrect for protracted periods, the neck muscles are unnecessarily stressed, causing discomfort that leads to headaches. Ergonomically, the body and eyes must be positioned in a way that is comfortable for the long term (see Chapter 5 for ergonomic tips). The proper prescription and lens design for the exact type of work being performed mitigates many ergonomic problems.

In addition to the normal positional constraints of using a computer, users of multifocal lenses are further restricted to even smaller movements of the eyes and posture to obtain clear vision while working. Computer or reading glasses prescribed for this specific task alone optimizes the reading area and alleviates the additional stresses placed on the eyes and the posture. A second pair of eyeglasses dedicated to near work pays handsome dividends in comfort, acuity, and productivity.

Acute Angle Closure

A rare condition called acute angle closure glaucoma is known to cause severe headaches and eye pain simultaneously. Acute angle closure is a medical emergency that requires immediate clinical treatment to prevent serious damage to the eyesight. The "angle" in the name refers to the anatomical drainage mechanism in the eye that discards old fluid. Some individuals are anatomically prone to having this drainage mechanism close down, which causes fluid to build up inside the eye and results in elevated intraocular pressure. An episode of acute angle closure typically presents with a very painful, red eye; cloudy vision; and frequently a headache. The pupil often becomes "fixed" and does not respond to light as it normally would. By measuring the elevated intraocular pressure and examining the closed drainage mechanism, an eye doctor can diagnose the problem and intervene to break the attack with a combination of topical and oral medications.

HEADACHES CAUSING EYE PROBLEMS

Many serious underlying health problems manifest with headaches occurring alongside other ocular symptoms. The eye is a window that sometimes provides doctors a view into other body systems. Inside the skull, the outer coverings of the brain extend out to also cover the optic nerve of each eye. Since the skull is not expandable, pressure from inside the skull may radiate down the optic nerve covering and cause the end of the nerve inside the eye to swell. Lesions that take up space inside the skull, such as a tumor, leaked blood from an aneurysm, inflammation from meningitis, or anatomical malformations, will cause intracranial pressure to increase, which may affect the appearance of the part of the optic nerve visible to an eye doctor. Optic nerve swelling can blur vision, which is one of the early symptoms along with headaches. Pseudotumor cerebri is a somewhat common condition that masks as a space-occupying lesion. Though no real tumor exists, severe headaches and optic nerve swelling do occur from increased intracranial pressure.

Medical observation of optic nerve swelling and a history of headaches will alert the doctor that further testing and imaging are necessary to determine if any of these serious underlying conditions are present.

Hypertension and Headaches

Undiagnosed high blood pressure may cause headaches and

blurred vision. If the hypertension is severe enough to cause headaches and optic nerve swelling, other ocular signs may also be present. In an individual with hypertension, the high pressure that exists inside the small blood vessels of the eye can rupture and spill blood. Multiple areas of retinal bleeding are often a sign to the eye doctor that undiagnosed hypertension exists. Eye doctors are equipped to test blood pressure and will refer the individual to his or her primary care physician (or an emergency room) if blood pressure is elevated. Once the blood pressure is brought under control, the headaches and ocular manifestations subside.

Ophthalmic Migraines

Migraine headaches occur in countless different forms and levels of severity. For many migraine sufferers, light sensitivity is a common symptom that appears with the severe headache. However, certain types of migraines affect vision far more profoundly than just light sensitivity.

Migraines of all types are brought on by a wide spectrum of unrelated causes. Common migraine triggers include extreme emotional or physical stress, hormonal changes, certain foods (including aged cheeses, monosodium glutamate, and red wine), lack of sleep, medications, and birth control pills, to name a few. Though not fully understood, migraines are thought to be caused by variances in blood flow to the brain caused by the dilation and constriction of intracranial blood vessels. If variances in blood flow also occur in the areas of the brain responsible for vision, visual disturbances related to migraines typically result.

Statistics vary, but it is believed that approximately 15 percent of migraine sufferers also experience ophthalmic migraines. Ophthalmic migraines cause alarming visual distortions or even temporary partial blindness in one or both eyes. A migraine visual aura is the episode of assorted visual disturbances that occurs just before a migraine headache. However, not all individuals who experience a migraine visual aura actually develop the headache after the aura. Migraine visual auras characteristically affect the eyesight for a period of approximately 15–60 minutes, after which vision returns to normal. The resolution of the visual changes can then usher in a severe, debilitating migraine headache for many people.

The initial visual symptoms of an ophthalmic migraine appear spontaneously and can be quite frightening. This is especially true during the first episode when a diagnosis has not yet been made. Symptoms vary among individuals and also fluctuate from one episode to another in the same person. The most common visual changes involve kaleidoscopic, colored sparkling lights in the peripheral vision; multi-colored zig-zag lines; arcs of flashing light; and blind spots in small or large areas of the visual field. The temporary blind spots are often centrally located, preventing the individual from looking directly at something. These are particularly terrifying if they occur while the individual is operating a vehicle.

People who have been previously diagnosed with ophthalmic migraines learn in subsequent episodes that the visual aura is a harbinger of an impending migraine headache, and they know to take medication immediately. Often the migraine headache can be avoided if over-the-counter (OTC) or prescription headache medication is taken immediately after the onset of the visual aura.

Some individuals suffer from an acephalgic migraine, also known as a "silent migraine." In my own experience, approximately 40 percent of the patients I examine with migraine visual aura symptoms do not experience any headache after the visual symptoms. Acephalgic migraines produce auras and other manifestations of a migraine episode, but do not cause the severe headache. It is imperative that an individual suspecting they have an acephalgic migraine still be clinically evaluated, as other non-migraine conditions such as high cholesterol, stroke, or retinal detachment may mimic the visual symptoms of a migraine visual aura without headache.

Treatment for a migraine visual aura is the same as for conventional migraine headaches. The most beneficial (but often most difficult) long-term treatment is to remove the migraine trigger. As we all know, this is often easier said than done, but behavior or diet modification are often very successful at reducing the number of migraine episodes. OTC analgesics such as ibuprofen (Advil) or naproxen sodium (Aleve), taken early in the headache episode, work well for many sufferers. Acetaminophen (Tylenol) may also provide relief. Caffeine taken at the same time as the OTC medication can work in concert to help alleviate the pain. Many OTC analgesics marketed to treat migraines already include caffeine as an ingredient, so make sure to check the medication label prior to consuming additional caffeine to self-medicate. If these measures fail to control the pain and disability, prescription oral or injectable migraine medications may be used to reverse the attack.

Migraine headaches and migraine visual auras do not typically cause any long-term damage to the eye or vision. Though the acute episodes of visual disturbances are debilitating and alarming, they are reversible and normal eyesight returns once the episode is complete. Migraine sufferers should be evaluated by their physician since other serious conditions, such as brain tumors, may mimic a migraine. In addition, people with migraines may unnecessarily suffer during an attack if they do not have access to the effective medications that exist today.

CHAPTER 12

SYSTEMIC DISEASE AND THE EYES

A number of systemic diseases can affect the health of your eyes and your vision. Here, we look at diabetes, hypertension, high cholesterol, and thyroid disease.

DIABETES MELLITIS

Diabetes is a disease that occurs when the levels of sugar (glucose) in the blood are not properly regulated. Glucose is the body's fuel, and levels need to be constantly regulated to provide the proper amount of fuel to keep up with the body's changing demands. The sugar levels in the blood are regulated by hormones. Insulin is a hormone that helps the body remove excess sugar from the blood and places it into storage for use at another time. Under normal conditions, our bodies constantly adjust the levels of sugar in our blood to allow the proper amount of "fuel" to reach muscles and organs. Insufficient or excessive sugar levels are problematic for the body, and diabetes revolves around this problem.

It is estimated that 8 percent of the U.S. population suffers from diabetes, and roughly 20,000 new cases of blindness due to diabetes occur each year. Approximately 30 percent of all diabetic patients have never had an eye examination. Fortunately, proper examination intervals and medical treatment decrease the incidence of blindness. Many cases of blindness due to diabetes could be prevented if an examination occurs early in the disease process.

There are two main types of diabetes: Type 1 diabetes is usually diagnosed during childhood and is caused by the body's inability to produce insulin. Type 2 diabetes is typically diagnosed in adulthood and is caused by the body's resistance to insulin, not from the lack of production. Diabetes variants share the same ocular manifestations regardless of the type.

Diabetes is the systemic disease most likely to also cause ocular disease, and nearly all parts of the eye are susceptible to damage from it. Every diabetic patient is at risk for ocular complications and should become educated about the potential risks. Diabetics who regularly follow up with their eye-care provider are in the best position to preserve their eyesight and to receive medical intervention before irreversible damage occurs.

Types of Diabetic Eye Disease

The retina is the part of the eye most commonly affected by diabetes. Diabetic retinopathy is the name for diabetic changes in the back of the eye, and there are several classifications: non-proliferative diabetic retinopathy (NPDR), proliferative diabetic retinopathy (PDR), and diabetic macular edema (DME). Diabetes is also associated with significantly higher incidences of glaucoma and cataracts. In addition, the external ocular muscles may be affected by diabetic disease and can cause improper eye movements that sometimes lead to double vision. Drastic daily fluctuations in visual acuity are common with high levels of blood sugar as well, and this can make normal daily functioning nearly impossible at times.

Diabetic Retinopathy

The main way diabetes is thought to cause damage to the eye is by excess levels of glucose abnormally affecting the pericytes, which are cells found in the small blood vessels of the eye. Pericyte damage is thought to be a primary cause of diabetic retinopathy, but it is not believed to be the only cause. In diabetes, the blood becomes thickened by excess sugar, and it develops a syrupy consistency. Imagine our blood vessels to be like a drinking straw. It is easy to suck water through a straw because water is so thin in consistency. However, trying to drink maple syrup through the same straw is significantly more difficult because of the viscosity (thickness) of the fluid. It is difficult for the thick, syrupy blood to pass through the smaller blood vessels in the eye, and sometimes the blood comes to a complete standstill rather than remaining in constant motion as it should. The thick blood can cause other blood components to leak out of the arteries and veins (exudation), and it may also cause small blood vessels to rupture and bleed. Retinal bleeding is one of the most common ocular manifestations of diabetes.

Another frequent complication of diabetes is neovascularization, or new blood vessel growth. Blood is the vehicle that carries oxygen to different parts of the body, including the retina. If blood flow to specific areas of the retina gets interrupted, the tissue that would normally receive its oxygen from that blood will suffocate. The body's answer to this problem is to grow new arteries to provide an alternate source of oxygen. While this seems helpful, the new vessels that grow are very weak and prone to rupturing and bleeding, which can be catastrophic to eyesight.

Early stages of diabetic retinal changes do not necessarily affect eyesight. However, findings such as small bleeds in the back of the eye are an early warning sign of more sight-threatening conditions. Even though the diabetic patient may be unaware of these small bleeds, their discovery in an eye examination can ensure earlier treatment. If intervention is not undertaken upon their detection, more serious ocular risks and complications are certain to occur. Undetected diabetic eye disease can be present and cause the patient no symptoms, then suddenly and unexpectedly, massive vision loss may occur. If the symptom-less early diabetic eye disease is diagnosed by a doctor, the impending sudden vision loss may sometimes be averted.

- Lower-Risk Diabetic Retinopathy: Mild and moderate levels of non-proliferative diabetic retinopathy may include small hemorrhages, changes to the appearance of the small retinal blood vessels, and exudation (the retinal accumulation of blood components outside of the blood vessels). These findings are sometimes limited to specific areas of the retina. The lower-risk findings are still cause for concern and may progress to more serious eye problems from diabetes. Lower-risk retinopathy does not normally pose an emergency level of threat to the eyesight. All therapeutic efforts to control blood sugar at these early stages of retinopathy must be made in order to prevent more debilitating vision problems from developing.

- Higher-Risk Diabetic Retinopathy: Severe NPDR and proliferative diabetic retinopathy *do* pose an immediate and high-risk threat of

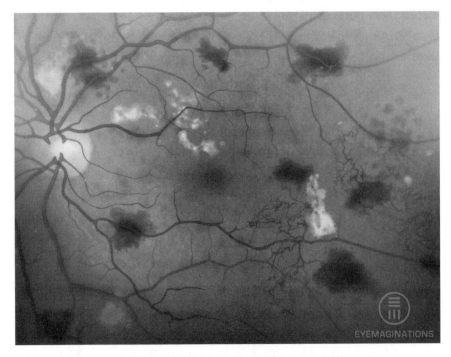

Diabetic Retinopathy

irreversible vision loss. Higher-risk retinopathy usually includes abnormal levels of bleeding, vessel abnormalities, and possibly neovascularization in all areas of the retina. Surgical intervention (discussed below) and tighter blood sugar control are typically the necessary steps at this stage.

Diabetic Macular Edema

Though macular edema is more commonly found in association with higher-risk retinopathy, diabetic macular edema can occur at any time and any stage of retinopathy. The macula is the most sensitive and visually important part of the retina. Swelling and edema (fluid accumulation) in the macular area is caused by leaky blood vessels, which are visually destructive. Typically, surgical laser intervention is necessary to prevent further blood vessel growth and bleeding in the macula.

Glaucoma

Diabetics have a 40-percent higher risk of developing glaucoma than non-diabetics. Glaucoma and diabetes are more commonly found in African Americans, who have a higher incidence individually for both glaucoma and diabetes. The odds of the two diseases being present together increase even further once the first one is detected. Glaucoma is a disease that occurs when the intraocular pressure increases to dangerous levels. The eye produces and drains fluid at a constant rate to regulate the pressure inside the eye. Diabetic patients sometimes develop new blood vessels in response to tissues not receiving enough oxygen. Unfortunately, new blood vessel growth may occur in the drainage mechanism of the eye and plug the drain. When the drain is blocked, fluid is retained in the eye, causing the intraocular pressure to rise. The rise in pressure can damage the optic nerve, which causes vision loss. At-risk patients are monitored by their eye doctor for the development of "neovascular glaucoma" as well as other types of glaucoma, since the association with diabetes is well known.

Cataracts

According to the American Diabetes Association, diabetics are at 60-percent higher risk for developing cataracts than non-diabetics person. While most people develop cataracts with maturity, diabetics tend to develop them faster and earlier in life than non-diabetics. In diabetics, cataract development may begin as early as their thirties and forties. Regardless of the presence of diabetes, wearing sunglasses whenever outdoors to protect against UV light may be partially effective against cataract formation.

Ocular Muscle Problems

Excess sugar in the bloodstream can cause imbalances in other body tissues, as well. If blood is restricted from properly reaching its destination to drop off the oxygen "payload," tissues may become damaged. Diabetics sometimes suffer from a reduction of oxygen reaching the nerves controlling the external eye muscles, causing eye tracking problems. The external eye muscles are responsible for our eye movements as we look in different directions. One of the most frightening manifestations of this symptom is an onset of double vision that may last for two or three months before resolving. An immediate medical evaluation is in order with the onset of any double vision. Though diabetes is a less severe cause of double vision, other serious underlying conditions causing double vision must be ruled out even for diabetics.

Fluctuating Vision

Diabetes is notorious for causing fluctuating eyesight and substantial vision prescription shifts. As blood sugar levels exceed 200 mg/dL, the physiological lens inside the eye collects additional sugar from the blood. The additional sugar in the lens draws fluid along with it, causing the lens to thicken. Just as thickening or thinning an eyeglass lens changes its refractive power, the same occurs in the diabetic eye: the fluctuating thickness of the eye's lens from hour to hour and day to day makes the eyesight constantly change. Undiagnosed diabetics with sustained high levels of glucose may present to their eye doctor with a complaint of fluctuating vision, and the doctor sometimes discovers that their prescription has doubled or more in power in a very short time. These two signs—large shifts in an eyeglass prescription during a short time and fluctuating vision—are often the first visual symptoms a diabetic will complain about. Typically, once diabetes is diagnosed and controlled, the blood sugar levels can be kept below 200 mg/dL to prevent fluctuating vision and other health complications.

Risk Factors for Diabetic Eye Disease

The most important risk factor in all diabetic conditions is blood sugar level. Undiagnosed or sustained, uncontrolled elevation of blood glucose levels are definitive causes of diabetic ocular manifestations. High blood pressure, high cholesterol, pregnancy, and cigarette smoking are all known to increase the risks of developing eye disease in people who are diabetic.

Not all diabetics develop ocular manifestations of the disease, but the risk increases proportional to the duration of diabetes. Even with excellent blood sugar control, many diabetics develop early forms of retinopathy after ten to fifteen years of the disease.

Testing for Diabetic Eye Disease

Diabetic eye disease—mild and even severe—can go undetected by an individual until there is acute catastrophic vision loss. The various stages of diabetic retinopathy rarely manifest in a way that immediately begins to affect the vision. Irreversible retinal damage may be underway for years before a diabetic person begins to question their ocular health or eyesight. The standard of health care today is for diabetic patients of all ages, races, and levels of disease to have a dilated eye examination performed by an eye doctor at least once a year. Both optometrists and ophthalmologists are trained in diagnosing and monitoring diabetic eye disease. Individuals who have ocular manifestations of diabetes will be advised by their doctor about more frequent examinations based on the particular findings.

The eye doctor will monitor the patient's refraction (eyeglass prescription) stability, external eye health, and internal eye health. Diabetes spares few ocular systems and also causes other ocular diseases such as glaucoma and cataracts. All of these will be evaluated during the eye examination. Microscopic evaluation of the iris, ocular fluid drainage system, and retina is critical for monitoring the development of diabetic eye disease.

Treatment of Diabetic Eye Disease

Proper diabetes management occurs when health-care providers across different specialties work together in a team approach to manage the disease. Primary care physicians, endocrinologists, eye doctors, dentists, and podiatrists are all involved in the total management of diabetes. The first line of treatment for any diabetic ocular manifestation is the coordination of treatment approaches between the eye doctor and the physician managing the systemic diabetes. Diet, exercise, and medical treatment of diabetes to control glucose levels are the only effective methods of preventing or forestalling the development of diabetic eye disease. Once diabetic retinopathy appears, medical treatments are available (limited but improving) to help control the vision problems.

Mild or moderate retinal bleeding may come and go without ocular treatment intervention in the early stages of diabetic retinopathy. Small retinal hemorrhages will resolve on their own as new ones appear, but the eye must be carefully monitored for hypoxia (lack of oxygen) so that new blood vessels don't develop, since these new vessels can rupture and spill blood, potentially causing blindness. If new blood vessel growth is present, various forms of laser eye surgery may be performed to destroy the vessels. Surgical lasers are used to cauterize the vessels or other selected areas of retina to stop new blood vessel growth in the eye. More severe surgical intervention may occur when blood has spilled and robbed an individual of eyesight. A vitrectomy (surgical removal of the vitreous fluid) helps remove the opaque spilled blood in hopes of restoring a clear path for light to reach the retina. Vitrectomy is delicate and risky procedure, but it is the only alternative to blindness that exists when diabetic eye disease has reached this level. While no treatments cure diabetic eye disease, surgical intervention can help keep the vision stable, and it usually deters progression for a longer period of time.

Glaucoma and cataracts associated with diabetes are treated essentially the same way as in individuals without diabetes. However, glaucoma treatment may need to be somewhat more aggressive than normal, and cataract surgery complications are increased in diabetics. The healing patterns of diabetics are more unpredictable, which affects the eye's ability to heal after surgery of any kind.

Double vision as a result of diabetes is primarily managed by better blood sugar control, but the eye doctor can help the patient cope with the temporary doubling by patching an eye or utilizing prisms in the eyeglass prescription. Fluctuating vision is controlled primarily through tighter blood sugar control as well. There is a direct correlation between blood sugar levels and eyeglass prescriptions. While eyeglass lenses can be remade over and over again, it is costly and inefficient since the eyesight may change as quickly as it takes to fabricate new lenses. Usually, the vision fluctuations are all but eliminated when blood sugar is well controlled.

Other than good glucose control, the top ocular health priority for diabetics is having an annual dilated examination by an eye doctor. Countless cases of blindness from diabetes can be prevented if the impending signs are diagnosed earlier.

HIGH BLOOD PRESSURE

Since high blood pressure and diabetes both affect the small blood vessels of the body, the eye is a place that is commonly affected by each of these conditions. The retinal changes that occur from both high blood pressure and diabetes often look the same to the eye doctor and can be differentiated only after blood pressure and blood sugar testing have been performed. The organ system most frequently associated in our minds with high blood pressure is the heart, but the eyes are sometimes the first place that undiagnosed hypertension is found. Hypertensive retinopathy is the name of findings in the retina associated with high blood pressure.

High blood pressure may never cause changes to the eye, but if it does it will be recognizable to your eye doctor. Hypertension infrequently causes blurry vision, but it is a possible cause when a doctor is evaluating the underlying cause of blurriness. It may cause the retinal blood vessels to become narrower and it is also known to cause areas of bleeding in the retina. Additionally, exudation (leaky blood vessels) and "cotton-wool" spots may be observed in the retina. As with diabetes, adequate levels of oxygen may not reach all areas of the retina because of hypertension, causing small patches of retinal damage. Because of their puffy, cottony appearance, these damaged areas are referred to as "cotton-wool" spots. More dramatically, hypertension may cause a "stroke" in the eye, resulting in non-reversible vision loss. A sudden, painless loss of vision in one eye may be a sign of a central retinal vein occlusion or a branch retinal vein occlusion precipitated by high blood pressure. With a retinal vein occlusion, areas of bleeding in the eye occur, affecting some or all of the retina. While victims of this kind of "stroke" may have recover some vision over time, most people are left with permanent visual reduction in the affected eye as a result.

There is no specific treatment for the eye itself when hypertensive retinopathy is present. The primary goal is to lower the blood pressure and prevent strain on the heart and kidneys. Upon diagnosing hypertensive retinopathy, the eye doctor will take a blood pressure measurement and direct the patient to the most appropriate care in a timely manner. Seriously elevated blood pressure may require an immediate trip from the eye doctor's office to the emergency room.

As blood pressure is brought under control, the ocular signs of hypertension usually improve. It is common for high blood pressure to be first diagnosed during an eye exam, but it is less common for hypertension to have lasting visual and ocular effects once systemic treatment commences.

HIGH CHOLESTEROL

Cholesterol is a lipid that makes up part of the body's microscopic cells, and it is a vital component for our health. Our bodies produce cholesterol, and we also ingest cholesterol through food. However, too much of a good thing leads to excess cholesterol in the bloodstream, causing significant health problems. Cholesterol is a sticky, waxy substance that is present in the blood. Excess cholesterol can adhere to the inside walls of the arteries and veins, which eventually leads to larger plaque formation. As these plaques form, the blood vessels become narrower, preventing blood from flowing well, much like a slow drain. A stroke occurs when a blood vessel becomes totally blocked by cholesterol build-up, preventing blood from passing through. Subsequently, the tissue downstream dies from lack of oxygen. Strokes can occur in the brain, heart, and eyes, depending on where the blood vessel blockage occurs.

Excess cholesterol can affect the eye in three different areas: the eyelids, the cornea, and the retina. Cholesterol deposits of the eyelids and cornea don't affect eyesight, but they indicate that more serious systemic problems such as undiagnosed high cholesterol may exist.

Xanthelasma

Cholesterol may accumulate in pockets just under the skin of the eyelids. Xanthelasma usually presents as whitish-yellow elevation on the upper and lower eyelids and brow area, typically closer to the nose. It is sometimes said to have an appearance resembling "chewed gum." Though the lesions don't affect vision, they are often a cosmetic concern and can be removed by a dermatologist or oculo-plastic surgeon. Xanthelasmas are known to be genetic, but their presence may indicate abnormally elevated cholesterol levels and warrant further blood testing.

Arcus Senilis

The most common ocular sign of high cholesterol is called arcus senilis, a white ring around the edges of the cornea in both eyes. Arcus is widespread throughout the mature population. It usually has no effect on vision or eye health, but it is a warning that levels of cholesterol in the blood may be too high throughout the body.

Eye doctors diagnose this ring around the cornea during a comprehensive examination and are prompted to question the patient about their cholesterol levels. While the presence of arcus does not always indicate high cholesterol, a strong correlation exists between the two findings. An even stronger correlation between arcus and high cholesterol exists when arcus is diagnosed in someone in their thirties or forties, as this is usually much too young to find cholesterol deposits in the cornea. Arcus senilis may become so dense—particularly in the elderly—that the white corneal ring is visible to the naked eye from a few feet away. Even when cholesterol levels are brought under better control through diet, exercise, and medication, the white corneal ring will remain. Once cholesterol deposits in the cornea, it remains regardless of overall blood cholesterol levels. Fortunately, this is not true for our arteries and veins, as proper treatment of the disease will remove excess cholesterol from the blood.

Hollenhorst Plaques and Ocular Blood Vessel Blockages

The great fear and concern with high cholesterol is that a blood vessel will become totally blocked by a cholesterol plaque. If blood is prevented from passing through arteries, oxygen is unable to reach the tissues downstream. If an entire organ system, or even part of an organ system, does not receive oxygen, it will likely shut down and die. Loss of vision, brain damage, and heart attacks are caused by lack of oxygen.

Cholesterol may obstruct large and small arteries alike. It takes longer for cholesterol to block a larger artery since the cholesterol plaque has a greater diameter to span before total occlusion. However, the health threat is immediate even if the entire vessel isn't completely blocked. Smaller pieces of an early plaque may break off and become free in the blood, allowing the "cholesterol chunk" to travel downstream. The free plaque will continue to travel through the arteries until it becomes lodged in a vessel smaller than the diameter of the plaque itself. This entirely blocks blood flow beyond the smaller artery, and tissue damage or death occurs downstream from that blockage.

The eye has numerous small arteries and is susceptible to blockage from small cholesterol plaques lodging in a retinal vessel. A cholesterol plaque stuck in a retinal artery is referred to as a Hollenhorst plaque. While this has serious implications for the eye, it is an even more serious indication of the poor state of overall health. A cholesterol plaque can cause blockage of the main artery supplying the eye with oxygen, or it may block an artery supplying only a small area of the retina. This unfortunately leads to immediate partial or total loss of vision. Some cholesterol plaques in the eye will break up and dislodge, causing only temporary visual disturbances.

Hollenhorst plaques of the eye are an uncommon finding. While coronary heart disease is the number one cause of death in the United States, problems from high cholesterol generally take a severe toll on other organ systems prior to severe damage of the eyes. Unfortunately, those who are diagnosed with retinal blockage from cholesterol have a high likelihood of death within several years of the diagnosis because of the pre-existing damage to other body systems. If levels of cholesterol are so high that an embolism has occurred in the retina, it is a forgone conclusion that other organ systems vital to life (heart and brain) are even more severely at risk. A complete medical work-up and treatment are vital if they haven't already occurred prior to the Hollenhorst plaque diagnosis.

Sources vary, but it is generally agreed that anyone over age twenty with a strong history of heart disease should have a cholesterol screening annually. Men and women without a family history should be screened annually beginning at about age thirty-five. Laboratory readings of high-density lipoprotein (HDL) cholesterol, low-density lipoprotein (LDL) cholesterol, total cholesterol, and triglyceride levels are obtained from a blood sample. Prescription drugs are very effective at lowering cholesterol levels, though diet and exercise modification are integral to proper regulation.

THYROID DISEASE

Thyroid eye disease is known by several names, including Graves' disease and Graves' ophthalmopathy. It is the complex of physiological changes to the eye and its associated tissues caused by abnormal levels of thyroid hormones, namely elevated levels (hyperthyroidism).

The thyroid is a butterfly-shaped gland in the lower neck. Several hormones are produced by the thyroid gland, but thyroid dysfunction may cause under- or overproduction of these hormones. Thyroid eye disease is usually the result of the overproduction of the T3 and T4 thyroid hormones. Women are more susceptible to thyroid problems than men, with statistics showing approximately one in fifty women experiencing thyroid dysfunction. Of those with thyroid dysfunction, only about 5 percent have manifestations that involve the eye. The onset of ocular symptoms related to hyperthyroidism is unpredictable and may occur well before, during, or long after the thyroid disease diagnosis and treatment.

Symptoms of Graves' Disease

Excessive thyroid hormone levels frequently cause inflammation in the eye socket but outside of the eye itself. The external eye muscles responsible for eye movements and the surrounding fat and tissues swell, which crowds the space in the eye socket. Since the socket is composed of rigid bone, there is no "give" to allow the swelling tissue to expand, and the eye is subsequently compressed.

The only direction that is not resistant to the swelling socket is where we see the eye. For this reason, the main symptom of thyroid eye disease is a forward-bulging appearance of the eyes called proptosis. An individual with proptosis appears to be "staring" all the time since the bulging eye forces the two eyelids to be open wider than normal. The crowded eye socket can cause considerable pressure, making the individual very uncomfortable.

Thyroid eye disease may result in the globe of the eye protruding so far that the eyelids are unable to fully close, leaving a horizontal band of the cornea constantly exposed to the air. The function of the eyelids is to spread moisture over the front of the eye each time we blink, but incomplete blinking due to the eyelids closing inadequately allows dryness to occur. Common symptoms of Graves' disease include scratchy and gritty eyes as a result of the dryness. Inflammation from the swollen tissues combined with dryness contributes to chronically, excessively red eyes.

Double vision may result from the abnormal function of the inflamed external ocular muscles. Since the range of motion of the external ocular muscles may be limited, proper eye tracking and binocular vision are hampered. The most serious symptom that Graves' disease may cause is loss of vision, including blindness. The optic nerve connecting the back of the eye to the brain occupies space in the eye socket and is susceptible to being compressed by the severe inflammation of the surrounding tissues. Swelling of the orbital tissues from Graves' disease may compress the optic nerve so forcefully that information is blocked from transmission between the eye and the brain, causing vision loss.

Treatment of Graves' Disease

Thyroid eye disease is managed by treating both the thyroid and the eyes. Thyroid-regulating medications, radiation, and thyroid removal are various methods used to manage the thyroid hormone imbalances.

The ocular symptoms of dry eye due to the eyes protruding are addressed with artificial tears and other methods of dry-eye treatment (see Chapter 7 for more information on dry eyes). In some instances, surgical tape may be used to keep the eyelids closed at night to preserve the moisture and health of the front of the eye. Sight loss may occur from severe drying of the eye, so it is important from both a comfort and a vision standpoint to keep the eye moist.

In cases of mild double vision related to Graves' disease, the eye doctor may have prisms ground into eyeglass lenses to eliminate the doubling. Severe cases of double vision are usually not helped by prisms and may require a surgical procedure called orbital decompression. This surgical procedure removes some of the fat surrounding the eye, some of the orbital bones, or both. The goal of the surgery is to create more room for the inflammation and to release the pressure on the eye and optic nerve. Only 5 percent of thyroid eye disease patients progress to a level severe enough to require orbital decompression. Some patients undergo orbital decompression strictly for cosmetic reasons to reduce the bulging of the eyes, but for others it is to preserve vision.

CHAPTER 13

SEXUALLY TRANSMITTED DISEASES AND THE EYES

A number of sexually transmitted diseases (STDs) can affect the eyes and cause vision problems. In addition, herpes viruses that are not sexually transmitted can also infect the eyes.

CHLAMYDIA

Chlamydia is the most common sexually transmitted disease in the United States, with estimates indicating approximately 4 million cases each year. *Chlamydia trachomatis* bacteria infect the mucous membranes, mostly affecting the sexual organs in both men and women. Many people with chlamydia have no symptoms. Chlamydia can infect the eyes, although this is uncommon in adults. Eye infections due to chlamydia are most common in newborns, transmitted when the infant passes through the birth canal of the infected mother.

Ocular Symptoms of Chlamydia

The most frequent ocular symptom of chlamydia (in the United States) is an eye infection that causes red eyes, accompanied by mucous discharge. Like other types of bacterial eye infections, the individual will complain of discomfort and the sensation that something is in the eye. Conjunctivitis due to chlamydia may last four or more weeks at time, whereas non-chlamydial infections resolve more rapidly, even without treatment. An eye doctor will check for other signs in addition to the redness and discharge. Often, the undersides of the eyelids develop bumps (follicles); additionally, collections of white blood cells ("infiltrates") in the cornea may be observed with a microscope. A simultaneous vaginal infection may also be a sign that the infection is chlamydia.

Trachoma is a far more severe stage of chlamydial eye infection, which can develop if the initial ocular infection is not treated. It is unusual to see trachoma in the U.S. because medications and access to care are so prevalent. However, developing nations, areas with poor sanitation, or areas with limited access to health care—including regions such as North Africa, India, and Southeast Asia—report more cases. Left untreated, the follicles under the eyelids continue to grow and flourish, which in turn rub and irritate the cornea on a chronic basis. The eyelids may "roll in," causing the eyelashes to constantly scratch the front of the eye, damaging its clear tissue, and the cornea may eventually develop scars that can lead to blindness when untreated.

Treatment for Ocular Chlamydia

Oral and ointment antibiotics, such as azithromycin and doxycycline, are widely available in developed nations. When taken for several weeks these medications are very effective at clearing the ocular infection caused by *C. trachomatis*. Provided that permanent scarring has not already occurred, the same antibiotics are also effective at treating trachoma. Similar oral treatment regimens are also used to treat vaginal chlamydia infections. Doctors discuss the best treatment options with the patient and will likely suggest that sexual partners be treated as well.

SYPHILIS

Like chlamydia, syphilis is a bacterial infection (caused by the spirochete *Treponema pallidum*) in men and women that is nearly always transmitted via sexual contact. It can also be transmitted to a newborn when passing through the birth canal of the infected mother. According to the U.S. Centers for Disease Control and Prevention (CDC), approximately one new case per 25,000 people was diagnosed in the United States in 2008, in addition to 430 babies born with syphilis. An estimated 45,000 people in the U.S. currently have various stages of syphilis.

Ocular Symptoms of Syphilis

Syphilis is called the "great imitator" because it is clinically challenging to diagnose. Syphilis shares symptoms with many other diseases, and the ocular symptoms of syphilis are no exception. Most structures of the eye can be adversely affected by syphilis, including the cornea, iris, pupil, and optic nerve. Syphilis infection is divided into several stages: primary, secondary, latent, and tertiary. The primary stage of syphilis may happen within the first three months of infection and can continue through the four stages over a period of many years. The last stages of syphilis infection may not occur until decades after the initial infection. It is uncommon in the U.S. to progress to tertiary syphilis because effective treatment is widely available.

The primary stage of syphilis is characterized by the presence of a chancre, a temporary, painless lesion that may occur on or inside various parts of the body, including the eyelid or on the white of an eye. Chancres are frequently found on the penis in syphilis. The chancre lesion normally resolves on its own after a few weeks and is not permanent.

Secondary syphilis can occur 1–3 months after the initial chancre and has more widespread effects on the eye than primary syphilis. In secondary syphilis, the eye may become red and inflamed for no apparent reason (episcleritis), the cornea may become inflamed (interstitial keratitis), and inflammation of the iris (iritis), retina (retinitis), and optic nerve (optic neuritis) may all be present at various times. The secondary stage ocular symptoms are not exclusive to syphilis. Since they have multiple other causes, the mere presence of these symptoms does not automatically lead to a diagnosis of syphilis.

Latent syphilis is a period of time without symptoms that may last for years, and the eye is also unaffected during this time. The final (tertiary) stage of syphilis may occur, causing severe symptoms including paralysis and blindness. Fortunately, the late stage of the disease is quite rare. A characteristic ocular sign of late-stage syphilis is an unusual pupil response called "Argyll-Robertson" pupil: the pupils do not constrict normally when presented with bright light, but the pupil constriction that normally occurs when viewing a close object remains intact. In addition to Argyll-Robertson pupils, all of the ocular symptoms possible in secondary syphilis may be present again in tertiary syphilis. Should syphilis go undiagnosed and untreated, the disease eventually results in death.

Treatment for Ocular Syphilis Symptoms

Systemic syphilis is treated fairly easily during the first year of infection using common antibiotics, such as penicillin. After one year of untreated syphilis infection, it is increasingly difficult to control. The ocular symptoms of syphilis have no special treatment outside of the normal treatment protocols used for the same conditions without underlying syphilis. Most ocular symptoms are treatable, particularly if the underlying infection is treated with antibiotics.

GONORRHEA

Gonorrhea is a bacterial infection (caused by *Neisseria gonorrhoeae*) in men and women that is nearly always transmitted via sexual contact. It can also be transmitted to a newborn when passing through the birth canal of the infected mother. According to the CDC, approximately one new case per 825 people was diagnosed in the U.S. in 2006. Approximately 700,000 people in the U.S. are estimated to be infected with gonorrhea. Gonorrhea bacteria thrive in warm, moist mucous membranes, including the eyes.

Ocular Symptoms of Gonorrhea

The main ocular symptom of gonorrhea is a severe eye infection called conjunctivitis. Bright red, painful, and pus-filled eyes are the hallmark symptoms of most bacterial eye infections, including gonorrhea. Gonorrhea conjunctivitis causes copious amounts of whitish-yellow discharge from the eyes that requires constant removal. The purulent discharge may mat the eyelids shut making it difficult to open the eyes without assistance upon awakening. Eyelid matting is also common in other bacterial infections, so lid matting does not necessarily indicate gonorrhea, but the amount of purulent discharge in the eye infected with gonorrhea may be excessive. If the infection goes untreated, especially in newborns, scarring can occur, which may permanently damage eyesight. Rapid treatment is imperative.

Treatment for Ocular Gonorrhea

Eye infections caused by gonorrhea are treated similarly to other types of bacteria-related conjunctivitis. Prescription antibiotic eyedrops are effective at curing the ocular infection, and oral prescription antibiotics are effective against infections in other areas of the body. As in all bacterial eye infections, the purulent discharge from the eye is contagious and may infect others. Proper hygiene is important during an active eye infection. Do not share towels, pillow cases, and washcloths with others, and wash your hands frequently.

Chlamydia infections can occur at the same time as gonorrhea, so the physician will likely test for both conditions when the first one is diagnosed. If treated early, ocular gonorrhea infections do not have long-term complications on eye health or vision. However, prolonged untreated eye infections may lead to scarring of the cornea, which may permanently impair vision.

PUBIC LICE

"Crabs" is a parasitic infection that affects pubic hair and other hairy body areas including the eyelashes. The pubic lice parasite (*Phthirus pubis*) looks like a crab under the microscope, hence the nickname. The parasitic infection occurs when the lice physically transfer from one person to another via close physical contact, usually sexual in nature. Approximately 3 million new cases of pubic lice are diagnosed in the United States each year, but the number of eyelash infections by pubic lice is much fewer. The medical name for lice eyelash infections is phthiriasis palpebrarum.

Ocular Symptoms of Pubic Lice

Itchy eyelids are the primary symptom of pubic lice infection of the eyelashes. The itchiness is sometimes accompanied by mild redness of the edges of the eyelids. The diagnosis of crab lice is made when the doctor observes the lice under a microscope. The nits (lice eggs) are usually found at the base of the eyelash, and can sometimes be seen with the naked eye upon close inspection. The lice may also be detected as they slowly crawl along the eyelashes. Because parents are in close contact with their children, the lice infection may innocently spread to children via towels, pillow cases, and clothing. However, when a child's eyelashes are infected with lice, it may be a sign of sexual exposure or abuse.

Treatment of Eyelash Infections by Pubic Lice

The number of active lice and nits present will help the doctor determine the best way to clear the eyelashes of the parasitic infection. The lice and nits can be individually removed from the eyelashes using surgical forceps, but this may be a lengthy process, and the nits are sometimes difficult to remove. Another treatment method is the application of ophthalmic ointment on the eyelashes—thickly coating the eyelashes with ophthalmic ointment will cause the lice to suffocate. The eyelids are then cleaned of the ointment and the lice after a few days. Effective commercial preparations for the treatment of head lice are available over the counter, but should *not* be used for treating eyelash lice. The head lice formulations are too harsh for the eyelids and will cause damage if they get into the eye.

HIV/AIDS

While HIV (human immunodeficiency virus) is not always transmitted sexually, it is common to become infected via sexual contact. The CDC estimates that approximately 1.1 million men and women in the United States have HIV/AIDS. HIV infection does not immediately lead to AIDS (acquired immunodeficiency syndrome), but may result in its development at some point. HIV attacks the body's immune system, and the gradual decline of immunity causes the body to become defenseless against disease and infections that would not normally threaten a healthy individual.

Ocular Symptoms of HIV/AIDS

There are several main ocular manifestations of HIV infection, though they may not occur in all people with HIV.

1. Chronically red eyes are common in patients with HIV. Various forms of corneal infection such as bacterial keratitis, herpes simplex keratitis, herpes zoster keratitis, and other forms of irritation cause redness. Uveitis, an inflammation of the tissue surrounding the eye, is also possible and causes significant redness and discomfort. Any unexplained redness of the eyes should be investigated by an eye-care provider.

2. Kaposi's sarcoma is a non-cancerous tumor that is sometimes found in HIV/AIDS patients. Kaposi's sarcoma lesions may occur anywhere on the body, including the eyes; however, skin lesions are more common than eye lesions. Ocular signs are a reddish-purple, non-painful bump that appears on the eyelid or on the whites of the eye.

3. Diseases of the retina secondary to HIV include the following:

- HIV retinopathy affects the retina similar to the changes from diabetes, including white, fluffy areas in the retina ("cotton-wool spots"), which come and go. In addition, small areas of retinal hemorrhaging develop and resolve on their own. In a minor percentage of patients with HIV retinopathy, oxygen is prevented from reaching the macula and may lead to blindness in the affected eye. This type of retinal disease is *not* due to new underlying infections setting in as a result of the reduced immune function.

- Cytomegalovirus (CMV) retinitis is the most serious eye disorder and affects up to 35 percent of all AIDS patients. CMV is nonsexually transmitted form of herpes virus. While it is estimated that 80 percent of all adults have antibodies to CMV (indicating that they were infected at some point), the immune system is normally strong enough to prevent the virus from becoming active. Herpes viruses reside dormantly in the body once the virus is contracted, but in people with compromised immune systems, CMV has an opportunity to become active. Once the virus reactivates, it can cause significant problems in the retina.

Symptoms of CMV retinitis consist of significant floaters in the vision, flashes of light, blurriness, or blind spots that have appeared. Active retinal inflammation from CMV may not necessarily produce any symptoms, but it is sight threatening nonetheless. Low CD4+ cell counts provide an opportunity for CMV to activate, so people with low counts should be examined by a retinal specialist every three months or more often. Blindness is not inevitable, but it is a risk due the possibility of macular damage or retinal detachments. CMV retinitis may occur in one eye or both, but eventually both eyes become involved.

Treatment of Ocular Disease Secondary to HIV/AIDS

- Depending on its source, the chronic redness may or may not be responsive to treatment. If active infection of the cornea or inflammation of the eye exists, treatment of the underlying cause with prescription eyedrops or oral medications will frequently resolve the problem.

- Kaposi's sarcoma lesions sometimes resolve on their own with systemic HIV medication treatment, or they may require chemotherapy treatments. In other cases, freezing the lesions, radiating them, or excising them is necessary. Doctors consider multiple factors when deciding the optimal treatment route.

- Non-infectious HIV retinopathy does not require any specific treatment for the eye. As oral medications to treat HIV are taken, and CD4+ blood cell counts improve, this type of retinal disease typically improves.

- Cytomegalovirus retinitis requires aggressive treatment to delay sight-threatening damage. While treatment does not cure CMV retinitis, it typically slows the progression. Antiviral medications such as intravenous Foscarnet or Gancyclovir are effective treatments.

A Word about HIV/AIDS Transmission

The HIV virus is known to be transmitted through sexual contact, the sharing of syringes (often in conjunction with illicit drug use), or rarely via blood transfusions. The virus may also be spread from a mother to child during birth or via breast milk.

Though low amounts of the HIV virus can be present in the tears of an infected individual, *tears have never been shown to transmit the HIV infection to another person.* While never recommended for anyone under any circumstances, sharing a contact lens between an infected and non-infected individual has never been proven to cause HIV transmission.

Scientific research does show that unprotected contact with HIV-infected blood is a likely route of transmission. As a strong precaution, open cuts and wounds should be protected from contact with HIV-infected blood or other body fluids.

NON-SEXUALLY TRANSMITTED HERPES VIRUSES

Not all herpes viruses are transmitted sexually—some are transmitted only via airborne particles or through contact with active herpes lesions. Herpes simplex virus (HSV) and herpes zoster virus (HZV) are the two main classifications of herpes. HSV can be further subdivided into types 1 and 2. Only HSV-2 is commonly associated with sexual transmission; the remaining non-sexually transmitted herpes viruses, HSV-1 and HZV, may have ocular manifestations.

HSV-1 characteristically affects the body "above the belt" on areas of the face, mouth, lips, and eyes. HSV-2 typically affects the body "below the belt" and can cause genital warts and lesions. HZV is responsible for chickenpox, shingles, and sometimes ocular manifestations as well.

Once you are infected with a herpes virus, it remains inside the body indefinitely. The virus reverts to a dormant stage of inactivity that is kept in check by the immune system. Sources of reduced immunity can allow the dormant virus to "reactivate" and make symptoms reoccur. Factors such as physical or emotional stress, lack of sleep, ultraviolet light, or illness may provide the proper conditions for the dormant virus to become activated. It is estimated that two-thirds of all adults have the dormant herpes virus in their bodies without any symptoms. Someone who had chickenpox as a child has the dormant HZV now.

Herpes Simplex Virus Type 1

HSV-1 is usually transmitted from one person to another via kissing or direct contact with an active herpes skin lesion. Though more common in adults, HSV-1 can be spread to children. An example would be when a parent with an active herpes lesion kisses their child. HSV-1 often causes cold sores to break out on the face, on the lips, or in the mouth. It may also cause a painful and dangerous lesion on the cornea. These skin and eye lesions occur when the dormant HSV-1 virus is reactivated, typically by some stressor.

Ocular Manifestations of HSV-1

HSV keratitis is an ulceration of the cornea caused by active herpes viruses "eating away" at portions of it. HSV keratitis may occur in isolation or in conjunction with an outbreak of cold sores around the mouth. This type of corneal attack typically occurs only in one eye at a time, though subsequent attacks may occur in the same or alternate eye. Each corneal attack episode increases the odds of a subsequent corneal infection by approximately 50 percent. After the initial episode of herpes keratitis, it may never occur again, but often it does recur in subsequent months or years if immunity is compromised.

HSV keratitis causes a very red and painful eye, often accompanied by light sensitivity, tearing, and decreased vision. If left untreated, the cornea may be permanently scarred and this can lead to blindness. Rapid and aggressive antiviral treatment of the corneal lesion typically controls the outbreak so that the cornea is restored to near-normal. The HSV-1 virus eats away at the cornea in a characteristically unique "dendrite" fashion, and optometrists and ophthalmologists are skilled at recognizing this diagnostic pattern. When the presentation is questionable, the doctor may have a laboratory culture the infection to definitively ascertain the cause.

Treatment of Ocular Manifestations of HSV-1

Prescription antiviral eyedrops and oral antiviral medications are immediately started to aggressively treat the outbreak. People with HSV keratitis are monitored very closely (some may even require hospitalization), especially in the initial few days, since the potential risk for loss of eyesight is high. It is not unusual for some corneal scarring to remain after the virus has been killed and the cornea has healed. The size, density, and location (central or peripheral) of the corneal scar dictates whether permanent visual changes will result.

Herpes Zoster Virus

HZV is not a sexually transmitted disease, but it can be transmitted by direct contact with a person with active lesions on their skin, or via airborne transmission through a cough or a sneeze. Though vaccinations now exist, chickenpox is a form of HZV that can be transmitted from one child to another via airborne transmission. The initial infection from zoster usually manifests as chickenpox and then goes into its dormant stage in the body. Though chickenpox rarely recurs, if the dormant virus is reactivated later in life, it usually manifests as shingles, a painful rash or streak of blisters that break out on the skin, typically somewhere on the torso or face.

Ocular Manifestations of HZV

The shingles rash may affect parts of the eyelid or the cornea itself. HZV is known to cause multiple problems with the eye, including superficial or deep corneal inflammation, inflammation of the tissue surrounding the eye (uveitis), or inflammation inside the eye at the retina or optic nerve.

Treatment of Ocular Manifestations of HZV

Each manifestation is treated differently, but most ophthalmic complications from zoster are treatable with analgesics to help reduce the discomfort, as well as steroids to reduce inflammation.

CONCLUSION

The turquoise-blue water of tropical ocean surf, fireworks, the Grand Canyon, the canals of Venice, Niagra Falls, and rainbows. Whether you've experienced these sights in person or just from photos, the wonder of their beauty is difficult to appreciate without eyesight. Nearly 80 percent of what we perceive through our senses comes via eyesight. Considering all that our eyes do for us, healthy eyes and vision are worth a little maintenance and prevention, and the use of first-rate optical correction devices.

The care of our vision and eye health is not necessarily difficult, but education and action are prerequisites to seeing well both today and in the future. The goal of this book is to help raise your level of awareness, but the action part is still up to you. Good eyesight is of critical importance and you can achieve it by numerous means, including by partnering with your eye doctor to devise a plan for your long-term ocular health. You already see perfectly, you say? As you've learned in this book, the eye is so much more complex and wonderful than just the metric of 20/20 vision. The eyes often give "danger ahead" signs well before eyesight is affected, so regular examinations are essential for preventing more serious problems down the road. Invest in your long-term health and vision—start now by making an appointment for an eye check-up.

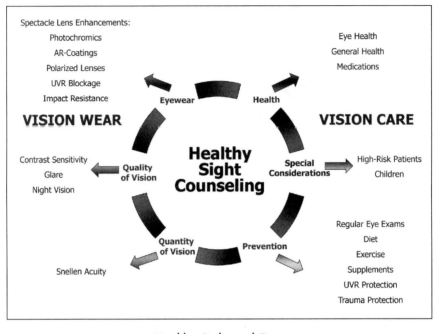

Healthy Sight and Eyes
© Transitions Optical, Inc. Reproduced here with permission.

Thank you for taking the time to learn more about your eyes. Your eyes thank you, too. I hope this book will serve as a reference to which you can return in the future as age-related concerns and other diagnoses potentially develop. I wish you and your loved ones a lifetime of healthy eyes and vision. Hindsight is 20/20, but no one said that your foresight can't be 20/20, too!

CONSUMER ADVICE ON VISION CORRECTION

EYEGLASSES

Frames

Eyeglass frames serve two purposes—function and fashion. Like clothing, eyeglass frame choices span the entire spectrum of price and quality. Also like clothes, eyeglasses are a reflection of the wearer's personality and tastes. Gone are the days when eyeglasses were something to be teased about. There are over 40,000 unique and current frame styles available for purchase in the United States, and many of them are branded by designers renowned in the world of fashion.

Fashion of Frames

From a fashion standpoint, some people are completely indifferent about their wardrobe, while others obsess over it. In general, though, we collectively want our clothes and eyewear styles to portray us in the most positive light. When we try on clothing, we opt for items that enhance our best features and hide our worst ones, and selecting eyeglass frames is no different. Right or wrong, the quality, overall condition, cleanliness, and designer logos of the clothes we wear silently impart messages to others, about our grooming habits, socio-economic status, tastes, and personality. If

Popular Brand Name Eyeglass Lines

Banana Republic	Donna Karan	Levi-Strauss
Barbie	Fisher-Price	Mont Blanc
Brooks Brothers	Giorgio Armani	Nautica
Calvin Klein	Gucci	Polo-Ralph Lauren
Chanel	Guess	Porsche
Disney	Harley-Davidson	Tommy Hilfiger
Donald Trump	Izod	Yves Saint Laurent

it is your style, wearing clothing that displays a designer's logo allows you to identify with that particular brand's "lifestyle." Designers spend millions of dollars each year to trigger specific images and feelings in our minds when we see their logo. Eyeglass manufacturers and designers know this and have shaped eyewear into a fashion accessory in addition to being a device for vision.

When choosing a frame, decide what your objective is in terms of appearance. The look and image you render can vary widely just by the frame you select. Do you want eyewear that is bold and colorful, playful and fun, or reserved and conservative? Do you want your eyewear to "pop" and stand out, or do you prefer eyewear that disappears on your face? Many people have several pairs of glasses to match their various moods. Eyeglass styles range from retro vintage up through modern, cutting-edge, haute couture designs. Do you have a favorite clothing line designer? Chances are they also have a complementary eyewear collection.

Function of Frames

Besides being fashionable, let's not forget the functional part that eyeglasses play, since they also enable us to see well. Eyeglass frames should hold your ophthalmic lenses in a stable position in front of your eyes for long periods of time, all while remaining completely comfortable. A well-fit frame should be both comfortable and light, eliminating the constant awareness of wearing eyeglasses, or the need to constantly readjust them on your face. Eyeglass frames touch our head in three places, over our nose ("the bridge") and over each of our two ears, so these are the areas to concentrate on when evaluating comfort. To improve the cosmetic appeal, frames that will be holding thicker lenses should be smaller in size and have a thicker eyewire to conceal lens thickness.

Metal or Plastic Frames?

Choosing between metal or plastic frames is largely a matter of personal taste. Various types of plastics and metals are used in the fabrication of eyewear. However, the material choice does affect the variables of comfort, durability, weight, and cost of the frames. When choosing frames, plastic material options are relatively similar. When choosing a metal frame, however, the base metal is a larger factor in the decision process. Most plastics are comfortable and durable, but metal frame characteristics vary widely. In fact, some metals react with sensitive skin and can cause a rash. Many metals are hypoallergenic, so if you have sensitive skin, make sure to mention it to your optician.

The most common type of plastic used in eyewear is called "zyl" (short for zylonite). This comfortable and durable plastic is available in limitless colors, so designers have a vast palate to work with. Zyl can also be laminated to produce attractive and colorful designs. Add those features to the nice luster possible after proper polishing, and you have the components that give plastic its timeless appeal for eyeglasses.

Metal frames are typically more durable than plastic, though not by a significant amount when considering quality eyewear. Metal frames can be alloys (combinations of various metals) or of a singular metal such as titanium. "Monel" is the most common type of metal used in the manufacture of eyeglass frames. Monel is a nickel alloy that is durable and provides good value. However, roughly 10 percent of the population is allergic to nickel, and a

Frame Anatomy

The frame front, also called the "eyewire," is the part that holds the lenses in place. Frame fronts are available in endless sizes, shapes, and colors. The area that connects the left and right eyewire as it crosses over the nose is called the "bridge." The function of the bridge is to support the weight of the front of the frame by resting on the nose. Since noses vary significantly, dozens of bridge designs exist to optimize the fit for differently shaped noses. Some bridges rest directly on the nose, and others are supported by adjustable nose pads.

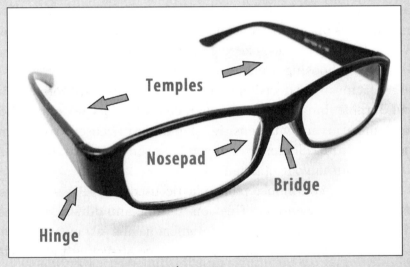

Eyeglasses Diagram

Many popular frame styles are "rimless" and have no metal or plastic around the lenses at all, but are instead constructed with direct anchor points where the bridge and ear pieces attach to holes drilled into the lenses. The metal components of a rimless frame style are called the "chassis."

The "temples" are the horizontal side pieces that hook over the ears. Temples stabilize the frame to prevent it from sliding down the nose and are adjustable to make the frame a custom fit. The temple is attached to the eyewire via a hinge so that the temples may be folded. Frame hinges are available in many different styles, some of them quite clever in design. Hinges are a "stress" point on the frame, so evaluating the hinge is a good indication of frame quality. Many frames have "spring hinges" that provide better frame durability and adjustment retention, but the quality of spring hinges can vary too. The most common shape of the temple-end is called a "skull temple" which bends slightly behind the ear. Other styles include "cable temples," which curve circularly behind the ear, and "library temples," which proceed straight over the ear without any downward bend. Opticians are able to precisely adjust the temples to customize the fit and comfort for each person.

small percentage of people develop a skin rash when wearing a metal frame containing nickel. Those with sensitive skin should look for plastic or hypoallergenic metal frames, such as titanium or aluminum.

Choosing a Frame that Compliments Your Face

While the following guidelines will help you narrow down your selection of eyeglasses, nothing beats trying on several frames to determine which one best compliments your face. Experienced opticians are skilled at evaluating facial features and skin tones to quickly narrow down which shapes look best so that you don't have to try on 500 frames to find the proverbial "needle in a haystack."

- Choose a frame shape that is the opposite of your face shape. If you have an oval face for example, try on rectangular frames.

- To size the frame properly, your pupil should line up behind the center of the lenses. If the frame is too big, your pupils will be inset from the center of the lens; if the frame is too small, the pupils will align outside the center.

- Choose a frame color that matches your skin tone and/or eye color for the most unified look.

Lenses

The lens materials and features you select are the starting point for a great pair of eyeglasses. It is a misperception that all ophthalmic eyeglass lenses are essentially the same. The quality and benefits of ophthalmic lenses vary substantially, and it is important to know what you are buying because it will affect your ability to see. Shopping for ophthalmic lenses can be confusing because there is an entire language used to describe lenses that is not part of the normal lexicon: *high index, progressives, index of refraction, UV-400, seg heights,* and other terms are often confusing. A higher-quality lens results in clearer, brighter, sharper, and more comfortable vision. Better quality lenses also increase the aesthetic appeal of eyewear.

Prescription eyeglass lenses of old had significant curvature on the front of the lens, which made them bulge outward from the frame. Newer lens technology has made it possible for virtually all prescription lenses to have a flat front surface (aspheric design). High-index lenses can now make once embarrassingly thick lenses extremely thin. Generally, as the lens prescription increases, so should the index of refraction to compensate for the high power. Polycarbonate and Trivex lenses are also very thin, strong plastics that are commonly utilized in prescription eyewear, and they are recommended for all eyeglass-wearing children under the age of ten. Police officers, firefighters, and other individuals susceptible to occupational or environmental hazards are usually prescribed polycarbonate or Trivex lens materials because of the built-in protection they provide.

Our eyesight is only as clear as the optics our eyes look through, and poor-quality optics can be a limiting factor in the clarity of our vision. When purchasing eyewear, you will need to decide on multiple lens options, each with its own substantial benefit. Depending on the retailer, these lens options are individually listed, or in some cases they are packaged together with the lenses. Since each person's needs are individual, lens choices are highly customizable.

Glass or Plastic Lenses?

The answer is plastic. Fewer than 3 percent of all eyeglasses manufactured in the U.S. are truly glass lenses; most are plastic for compelling reasons. Most ophthalmic lens manufacturers have stopped producing glass lenses, because plastic lenses are more scratch resistant, lighter weight, and more impact-resistant than glass. Until the 1980s, glass lenses were thought to have better scratch resistance than plastic lenses. Since then, the scratch-resistance technology of plastic caught up to glass and has now far exceeded the durability of a glass lens.

Scratch Resistance

No lens is entirely scratch proof, but the scratch-resistant lens treatments available are amazingly durable. The best-quality lenses can even withstand steel-wool abrasions, though I don't recommend that you test this! Lens scratches are detrimental because they scatter the light entering the eye, substantially degrading eyesight by inducing glare, shadows, or even double images. The additional glare caused by scratches is bothersome above all when driving at night.

Scratch resistance is an area that broadly varies in terms of quality among optical retailers. The best way to accurately ascertain whether a scratch-resistant lens is going to be durable is by scrutinizing the warranty behind it. Scratch warranties vary from periods of three months to two years, with the longer warranty found on the best-quality lenses. Inquire whether the scratch resistant treatment is on both sides of the lens or just the front surface, as the lowest-priced scratch-resistant lenses have the treatment applied only to the front.

Non-Glare Lenses

Also known as anti-reflective lenses, this feature delivers two benefits. Lenses with a non-glare treatment allow more light to the eyes, and the lenses look more aesthetically pleasing as well. Without the non-glare feature, eyeglass lenses pass through approximately 92 percent of the incoming light to the eye; the other 8 percent of light is reflected off the lenses. The front surface of the lens, the rear surface of the lens, and internal lens reflections mirror some of the incoming light, causing an overall reduction of light transmission. Proper illumination is critical for optimizing visibility, and it becomes even more critical in visually compromising conditions, such as driving in the rain. Computer users benefit from better contrast with non-glare lenses and suffer less eye fatigue. A high-quality, non-glare lens treatment will reduce virtually all glare and make the eyeglasses look as if there are no lenses in them, because they reflect little to no light.

Cleanability and Smudge Resistance

The highest-quality lenses and non-glare treatments offer better smudge resistance and cleanability. Quality optical lenses are treated with a hydrophobic agent that repels skin oil, dust, and debris from settling on them. Rather than streaking when they are cleaned, or easily showing the oil from our face or fingers on the lenses, the hydrophobic lenses are more user friendly.

High-Index Lenses

The purpose of a corrective eyeglass lens is to bend (refract) light into proper focus on the retina. A highly nearsighted or farsighted person needs his or her eyeglasses to bend light a greater distance than someone with a lower prescription. The *index of refraction* is a measure of how quickly a clear substance bends light. Images of thick, bulky, and unsightly lenses are often conjured when discussing a high prescription. However, modern lens materials allow lens fabrication with denser plastics that bend light faster, resulting in much thinner and lighter lenses. A high-index lens gets the job done with a reduced amount of lens mass and thickness.

Today's high-index eyeglass lenses are up to 70 percent thinner than similar lenses a decade ago. Because the lenses are thinner, a number of the optical aberrations induced by thick lenses are mitigated as well. There are many indices of refraction to choose from when purchasing eyewear, and the lens cost increases with the index. Someone with a moderate prescription who wants to benefit from a thinner and lighter lens doesn't have to buy the most expensive and highest index lens on the market. A knowledgeable optician can tailor the most cost-effective index lens to each individual.

Photochromic Lenses

Photochromic lenses are lenses that are clear indoors and darken to a tint outdoors. There are several brand names of photochromic lenses on the market, the most well known being Transitions®. Photochromic lenses are a popular option since they allow a single pair of eyeglasses to function as both a clear ophthalmic lens and as sunglasses. A heat and ultraviolet light-sensitive chemical in the matrix of the lens microscopically changes shape and causes the lens to darken with these stimuli. Each new generation of photochromic lenses gets lighter indoors and darker outdoors than the previous generation. Now, the lenses are so clear indoors that it is virtually impossible to see any residual tint, and they are extremely dark outdoors.

The only drawback that technology has yet to overcome is that photochromic lenses will not darken when used inside of a car. All front windshields of automobiles have an ultraviolet (UV) filter built in to prevent the dashboard from discoloring and cracking due to extended sun exposure. UV exposure to the front of a photochromic lens is necessary to cause them to darken, but windshields prevent UV from reaching the eyeglass lenses. Knowing this, many people still purchase photochromic lenses for their everyday convenience, yet also have a separate pair of prescription sunglasses for the car.

Multifocal Lenses

After the age of forty, most people need more than one prescription to see clearly at all distances. Presbyopia, the diminishing ability to see near objects clearly, usually necessitates a separate prescription from the one used for distance. Multifocal lenses are the solution to this problem for many people. As the name implies, multifocal lenses provide multiple focal points ranging from reading distance to far away.

When looking five feet away or farther, our eyes line up parallel to each other, and when reading or looking at a computer, our eyes turn inward and down. A multifocal lens is designed so that the distance prescription is situated in front of the eyes when looking far away, and the near lens prescription is located in front of the eyes when we look down and inward.

Lined Bifocals and Trifocals

Most everyone has seen eyeglass lenses with horizontal lines in them. This design has been available for hundreds of years and is known as a "flat-top" bifocal or trifocal. These practical lenses give the user a large field of view through each segmented lens prescription. However, they do have drawbacks both functionally and cosmetically. It is not normal for our eyes to have harsh lines in front of them. Optically, there is a "jump" the eyes go through when they make the vertical transition between multiple lens segments. Our eyes are accustomed to a gradual shifting of focus between different depths of field, and there is nothing gradual about flat-top lenses. A new user of flat-top lenses adjusts to this design after just a few days, but it never feels completely normal. Also, many people dislike "advertising" the implied stigma of maturity by wearing a lens with a line that everyone can see.

Progressive Lenses

Since the 1970s, lens technology has evolved to provide an improved multifocal lens option frequently referred to as a "no-line" bifocal.

These lenses house multiple prescriptions like a lined flat-top lens does, but there are no visible lines. Rather, they "progressively" change in prescription as the eyes view lower down in the lenses. Progressives more closely mimic our normal eyesight because they provide clear vision at any distance without inducing a "jump" between prescriptions. Plus, progressive lenses cosmetically look just like a single prescription lens, so no one can see that the user has a multifocal lens.

Progressive lens technology does not yet allow completely clear horizontal fields of view at the intermediate and near prescription ranges of the lens. Progressive lenses are like an invisible hourglass in their lens design. The top half of the lens is very wide, providing a wide useable area for the distance prescription that fully extends from one edge of the lens to the other. As the user views lower into the lens channel to the intermediate distance prescription (19–25 inches away), the horizontal field of view becomes narrower like the narrowest part of an hourglass. Then the reading area widens again when viewing even lower into the lens that focuses 14–18 inches away.

In the world of optics, progressive lenses probably have the widest spectrum of variation in quality. The lowest priced progressive lenses are less than $100 per pair, and the most expensive progressive lenses in boutique optical shops are approximately $700; most high-quality progressive lenses fall in the $300 to $400 range. Why such a difference in price? Clarity of optics, ease of adaptation and use, increased visual comfort, and customized optics are all answers to that question. While price is a factor that should be considered, the value of progressive lenses should be calculated by how well you see.

Learning to use any type of multifocal lens can take a short period of time. A primary concern is walking down stairs. Standing at the top of a staircase, we look through the lower part of the eyeglass lenses to view the first step down. With a multifocal, looking through the lowest part of the lens focuses our eyes 16 inches in front of us, not several feet away at the steps. Without proper

Buyer Beware

As the old adage says, "You get what you pay for." Quality optical frames and ophthalmic lenses start with the best raw materials. The base eyeglass lens is the foundation that any additional lens treatments are added to, so the quality of the optical system is limited by the weakest link in the optics. Choosing high-quality lenses will repay dividends on your investment in the form of clearer, more comfortable eyesight, and longer service life of the eyewear. Superior craftsmanship, durability, and customer service contribute to the cost of any optical product. Like any product, low-quality raw materials, shortcuts in craftsmanship, and looser tolerances are ways manufacturers can cut corners to reduce costs. Most optical retailers are trustworthy sources of information and products, but some less-than-scrupulous behaviors and vendors exist in the optical industry just as in other industries.

Optical retailers compete on the same three selling points that most retailers do: price, quality, and service. It is difficult, if not impossible, for a retailer in any industry to be the best at all three simultaneously. Most consumers aren't familiar enough with the optical industry to confidently make fully informed decisions about their eyewear selections without some assistance. However, everyone understands the common denominator—money—so cost is sometimes the only factor consumers consider when choosing eyewear. Optical retailers are aware of consumers' relative ignorance about optics, so some discount optical establishments make price their main competitive edge. Other retailers focus on educating their customers about the superior-quality products and put a bigger emphasis on customer service. There is room and demand in the marketplace for all types of retailers to exist, and you need to decide which qualities are most important to you when shopping for eyewear.

Inferior-quality eyewear will bite you back: the frame finish and color will often tarnish or fade; the hinges and screws may be weak, breaking easily with normal use; and cheap nosepads make the eyeglasses uncomfortable to wear for extended periods of time. Low-quality frames won't hold their adjustments and can diminish the optics. This is particularly a problem with multifocal lenses. You don't have to buy a designer brand to get high-quality eyeglasses, but they are generally a good assurance of quality. Well-known brands won't risk diminishing their reputation by putting their label on an inferior product.

When economics allow, using a reputable retailer to buy good-quality optical products is a safe bet. How do you find a trustworthy optical retailer? The same way you find a reputable doctor —by word of mouth. Ask friends and co-workers who wear eyeglasses about their experiences. When you see someone wearing an attractive pair of eyeglasses, don't be afraid to ask them about where they bought them. Rarely is a person bothered by receiving a compliment on the way they look in their eyeglasses.

vigilance, safe footing while descending the stairs can be easily misjudged unless the head is tilted down to look at the stairs through the distance part of the lens.

When looking at the computer or closer to read, progressive lenses have small peripheral "dead" areas that do not provide usefully clear vision. Better quality lenses mitigate these undesirable zones but can't eliminate them altogether. Walking while wearing progressive lenses and looking down to the side can cause a small amount of "swim" distortion, and it may take a few days to adjust to this. Most people who purchase high-quality progressive lenses adapt to them very well after a few hours or days.

CONTACT LENSES

Nearly 10 percent of the U.S. population wears contact lenses. Contact lenses are a safe, comfortable, and convenient vision-correcting option that is affordable to most people. Contact lenses correct most vision prescriptions for nearsightedness, farsightedness, astigmatism, and even multifocals. Because contact lenses rest on the eye's living tissue, and the risk of unmanaged complications can be sight threatening, they are available only by prescription.

Contact lenses have several advantages over eyeglasses. Contacts correct vision without anyone else seeing the lens, they don't fog up or get knocked off the face, and they provide better peripheral vision than eyeglasses. Optical aberrations and distortions induced by eyeglass lenses are reduced or eliminated with contacts, particularly with higher prescriptions. Some contact lenses are approved for overnight wear, so the benefit of being able to see well immediately upon awakening is available for many people.

Dozens of manufacturers make contact lenses, with the four largest U.S. companies being Coopervision, Ciba Vision, Bausch & Lomb, and Johnson & Johnson/Vistakon. If you wear soft contact lenses, chances are one of these companies makes your lenses. Nearly 90 percent of contact lens wearers use soft contacts, and the remaining use rigid gas permeable lenses (RGPs). Soft contact lenses are relatively inexpensive, very comfortable, convenient, and healthy options when worn as prescribed. RGPs provide exceptional optics and clarity of vision, but require more work to initially fit and adjust to. However, RGPs are less expensive than soft lenses on an annualized cost basis.

Maintenance and Replacement

Manufacturing efficiencies have permitted contact lenses to be mass produced for a relatively small cost compared to other optical devices. Just like putting on fresh clothes each day, it is healthier and cleaner to replace contact lenses on a regular basis. Gone are the days when one pair of lenses is maintained for a year at a time by boiling, cleaning, and soaking them with multiple agents to make them endure. Quarterly, monthly, bi-weekly, and daily replacement contact lenses are all popular today. Unless directed differently by the prescribing doctor, most disposable contact lenses don't even require rubbing to clean them. Simply by soaking them overnight in an "all in one" contact lens solution, the lenses will remain clean for the duration of the replacement interval.

The most important maintenance requirement for a contact lens wearer is an annual examination by an eye doctor, so that the health of the cornea can be monitored. Overwear or misuse of contact lenses can have serious consequences, including blindness. Early and sometimes subtle signs of impending problems are often first detected by the doctor during an exam.

Overnight Wear—Is It Safe?

Being able to see well 24-7 is a dream come true for most nearsighted and farsighted people. Especially when high prescriptions are involved, it may be difficult for an individual to even walk from the bedroom to the bathroom in the middle of the night without first reaching for their eyeglasses. The convenience and safety of being able to see well at all times without the fuss of eyeglasses has made overnight wear of contact lenses (and laser eye surgery) very attractive to many people. Parents with newborns waking up multiple times a night, emergency responders, and those who live alone feel safer having clear vision from the moment they open their eyes.

Oxygen transmission to the eyes via contact lenses is a critical factor in the short- and long-term health of the eye. Most contact lens-related complications are caused by a lack of oxygen reaching the eye. Newer contact lens materials, specifically the silicone-hydrogel class of contact lenses, are more oxygen permeable compared to older lenses from just a few years ago. Ciba Night & Day and Bausch & Lomb PureVision brands are both very permeable silicone-hydrogel lenses that have U.S. Food and Drug Administration (FDA) approval for up to thirty days of continuous wear. These lenses are considered safe for overnight use when properly fit and monitored by an eye doctor, provided the lens replacement schedule is followed and the cornea is monitored for ongoing health. Other silicone-hydrogel lenses prescribed today have six-night extended wear approval, even though most users still take them out each night before bed.

For a brief time in the early 1980s, the FDA approved several contact lenses (less permeable than today's standards) for overnight wear, but then quickly retracted it because a large number of ocular complications were reported. Subsequently, the public and eye doctors alike became distrustful of overnight-wear contact lenses. However, today's continuous-wear lenses have been on the market since 1998 without any widespread problems. Complications typically crop up as a result of people overwearing them or being non-compliant with their doctor's instructions. Most complications are minor and are resolved without consequence, but serious and sight-threatening problems are possible. After all, the lenses are in the eyes for a longer time, potentially exposing the wearer to higher risk of inflammation and infection—the two most prevalent concerns with contact lenses. Various durations of overnight wear reveal different statistics, but complication rates for microbial infections related to overnight wear range from 1 to 15 out of every 10,000. The largest fear is the rare but potential development of a corneal ulcer that leaves a permanent scar.

Every eye doctor has their own opinion and comfort level with fitting patients in overnight-wear contact lenses. With proper education and compliance, most people can safely use approved contact lenses for overnight wear. I personally have alternately worn the PureVision and Night & Day contact lenses on a one-month continuous schedule for several years without problems or apprehension. If you are interested in wearing overnight contact lenses, start by having a discussion with your eye doctor about the benefits and risks specific to your eyes.

Ocular Risks of Contacts

When used and disposed of properly, contact lenses have proven to be very comfortable and healthy on the eyes. However, inflammation, lack of oxygen, and infections are potential complications from contact lens wear. With the advent of disposable contact lenses in the 1980s, the number of complications from contacts dropped precipitously. Improper hygiene and lens overwear are the root causes of most complications. Since contact lenses generally still grant clear and comfortable vision beyond the recommended replacement schedule, many people falsely assume they are wisely saving money by stretching the lenses beyond their prescribed life. While this does in fact save money on the lenses, it is a false economy because the potential long-term vision problems can be far more costly.

All of our body's tissues need oxygen, and oxygen is delivered to tissues by blood traveling through arteries and veins. The cornea is a clear tissue that permits light to enter the eye, so it has no arteries and veins. Rather, the eye gets its oxygen from the fluid behind it and directly from the air. Contact lenses allow oxygen to pass through them to reach the cornea, but they don't transmit as much oxygen as possible without a lens. As the contact lenses age, proteins present in our tears deposit on the surface of the lenses, as well as in the microscopic pores that normally let oxygen pass through the lens. The prescribed replacement period of each lens is based on its unique oxygen permeability characteristics and its resistance to protein buildup. Reduced oxygen transmission by the lens does not affect comfort or vision, but it can cause an acute, sight-threatening condition without any warning. These painful and sometimes debilitating inflammatory and infectious responses may be severe enough to cause blindness. This is hardly worth the risk, considering the relatively minor costs of replacing the lenses as prescribed.

Buying Contact Lenses

With a valid prescription, contact lenses are available for purchase from the prescribing doctor, online stores, "big-box" retailers, and some pharmacies. When there is no differentiation in lenses regardless of where they are obtained, the first thought is to purchase from the source with the lowest cost. However, cost is not the only factor to consider when purchasing contacts.

Historically, contact lenses were available only through a doctor's office. As mass merchandisers and online retail gained market share, their bulk purchasing power allowed them to sell contacts at a lower cost. Now, all contact lens suppliers sell similar products competitively within a small price range, though some exceptions of wider variation still exist.

Many doctors' offices and retailers stock inventory of the most frequently prescribed brands and powers of lenses for immediate dispensing, but the sheer number of options makes it impossible for even the largest distributors to carry every lens. Often, lenses need to be ordered and can be shipped directly to the buyer, regardless of the source from which they are purchased. Contemporary eye-care practices compete equally with the convenience and price of the online retailers and offer direct shipment of contact lenses via their own practice websites.

When ordering from an eye-care practice, you receive better assurance that you will get exactly what your doctor prescribed. Free replacements of torn or defective contact lenses are also easily processed via a local doctor's office, but most mass merchandisers do not make allowances for this. Another concern people have is what to do when they've purchased a year's worth of contact lenses only to find their prescription changes before they've depleted their supply. While many vendors do not allow returns, most eye-care practices do.

LASER EYE SURGERY

Refractive surgery is the family of surgical procedures intended to correct for nearsightedness, farsightedness, astigmatism, or presbyopia. First pioneered in the 1970s, radial keratotomy (RK) was a method of surgically applied relaxing incisions to the cornea, which flattened its shape. RK was performed with varying degrees of success, but it opened the door to the possibility of new technologies in correcting vision problems. In 1995, the FDA approved a laser-based refractive surgical procedure called photorefractive keratotomy (PRK). PRK is still performed today, but the most common laser vision correction procedure now is LASIK.

LASIK was approved by the FDA just a few years after PRK. Both are somewhat similar in technique, differing only by how the laser ultimately accesses the layer of cornea intended to be modified. The PRK procedure reshapes the cornea after a surgeon scrapes the outermost layer of corneal cells (a painless procedure) in preparation for the laser. The outermost layer then grows back during the weeks after surgery. LASIK, however, is applied to the cornea after a re-positional flap of corneal tissue is surgically created. Folding the flap open allows the laser to gain access to its intended destination, and then the flap is returned to its closed position.

LASIK is superior to PRK in both the desired visual results and healing rates, but both enjoy similarly high success rates. However, PRK is a more flexible option for certain people who do not qualify for LASIK. Both laser surgeries are outpatient procedures—in

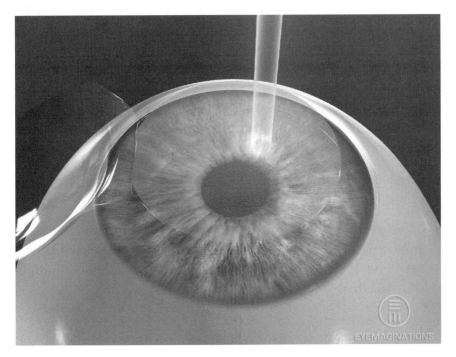

LASIK Application

fact, the actual surgery takes less than ten minutes, with the laser application taking only seconds.

Over 17 million refractive surgeries have been performed worldwide, with 8 million in the United States. In the late 1990s, it was thought that laser surgery technology would eventually herald the extinction of eyeglasses and contact lenses, but the statistics tell us a different story. While outcomes of laser eye surgery are safer and better than ever, the number of procedures peaked at about 1.4 million in 2000 (approximately 700,000 people). Between 2005 and 2009, laser surgery procedures steadily declined; only about 1 percent of the market (fewer than 500,000 people in 2009) needing vision correction chose laser surgery. Factors other than safety are likely to blame for the decline in popularity, not the least being the worldwide economic crisis that started in 2008. Since insurance companies do not pay for elective surgeries such as LASIK, the cost is entirely shouldered by the patient.

Despite the declining popularity, laser vision correction remains a viable and safe alternative to eyeglasses and contact lenses. Recent surveys reported that nearly 90 percent of vision correction surgery patients recommend it to others. When surveyed after surgery, 70 percent of LASIK patients said they felt "amazed and delighted" with the results.[16]

A few things you should keep in mind about laser vision correction:

- If you have laser surgery, the likelihood of needing reading glasses over the age of forty is still nearly 100 percent.

- Choose a reputable, experienced surgeon. An optometrist who doesn't perform the surgery but has examined many people who have undergone the procedure can be a great unbiased opinion when evaluating surgeons.

- Ask the surgeon what other costs to expect outside of the surgery itself, including follow-up visits, post-operative eyedrops, and potential enhancement ("touch-up") procedures in the future. The total cost of laser surgery from a reputable surgeon with the latest technology remains at about $2,000 to $2,500 per eye.

- Don't buy the least expensive "parachute," or laser eye surgery, that you can find. Cutting quality in these areas can be devastating.

Should I Have Laser Vision Correction?

Only you can answer that final question after you have been cleared by a surgeon to proceed, but you must first meet certain criteria to be safe. Eye doctors don't want you to have a poor outcome any more than you do, so "borderline" cases are rejected as candidates for surgery. If a surgeon gives you the disappointing news that you do not make a good candidate for laser surgery, I would not recommend investing a great deal of time searching for a surgeon who will give you an alternate answer. Candidates for laser surgery are qualified based on two broad categories: medical qualification and expectational qualification.

From a medical standpoint, good candidates for laser surgery need to have otherwise healthy eyes pre-operatively. Patients with moderate to severe glaucoma or any diabetic manifestations are poor candidates for laser vision surgery. Dry eye is a potential chronic side effect of laser surgery, so patients with pre-existing dry eye are counseled about this, and may be completely ruled out for surgery. Adults who have matured beyond expected growth spurts with a stable eyeglass prescription of at least one year are best suited for the procedure.

Eye doctors also attempt to ascertain the patient's motivation for and expectations of the surgery to make sure they are in alignment with reality. Though harder to quantitatively measure, eye doctors also attempt to evaluate each patient's "blur" tolerance. Certain individuals are more "visually sensitive" than others, and those with exceptionally high visual demands are more apt to be disappointed with the results of laser surgery.

Alternatives to Laser Eye Surgery

Besides the obvious alternative of eyeglasses, several other alternatives to laser eye surgery are available. With the advent of extended-wear contact lenses, many people once interested in surgery have fallen back on the familiar option of contact lenses. Unlike surgery, which can't be undone, high-oxygen lenses offer a less expensive and reversible alternative for 24-7 clear vision.

Another alternative is corneal reshaping. Ortho-Keratology lenses are worn overnight and removed during the day. These highly customized rigid gas permeable lenses gently and temporarily reshape the cornea while the wearer is sleeping. Since the cornea retains its temporary shape for 24–48 hours, users can remove the lenses while awake and still have clear vision. This temporary corneal reshaping lasts only as long as the contact lens is used and will revert to the original shape upon discontinuation (see Chapter 3 for more information on Ortho-Keratology). However, corneal reshaping may not be an alternative for everyone, and laser surgery corrects a broader range of prescriptions.

Intraocular lenses used for cataract surgery are also an alternative to laser eye surgery, even if the individual doesn't have cataracts. Called a "clear-lens exchange" without the presence of cataracts, implantable lenses can compensate for nearly all prescriptions. Not all refractive surgeons offer this option, but clear lens exchange is a well-tested and low-risk surgery. However, nearly all individuals undergoing clear lens exchange will require reading glasses after the operation, regardless of age.

Your eye-care provider can be a trusted source of information to discuss all vision-correction options. It is helpful to consider your visual goals and underlying motivation for seeking alternatives to the vision-correcting methods you are using. This will help you and your doctor customize alternatives best suited to your objectives.

REFERENCES

1. Chiang, Y., L.J. Bassi, J.C. Javitt. "Federal Budgetary Costs of Blindness." Millbank Q 2 (1992): 336-337. American Optometric Association (AOA). "AOA Optometric Clinical Practice Guideline, Comprehensive Adult Eye and Vision Exam Pamphlet." Alexandria, VA: American Optometric Association, 2009.

2. Christen, W.G., R.J. Glynn, A.A. Umed, et al. "Smoking Cessation and Risk of Age-Related Cataract in Men." *JAMA* 284 (2000): 713–716.

3. Targher, G., M. Alberiche, M.B. Zenere, et al. "Cigarette Smoking and Insulin Resistance in Patients with Noninsulin-Dependent Diabetes Mellitus." *J Clin Endocrinol Metabol* 82:11 (1997): 3619–3624.

4. Solberg, Y. "The Association Between Cigarette Smoking and Ocular Diseases." *Survey Ophthalmol* 42:6 (1998): 535–547.

5. Mutti, D.O., G.L. Mitchell, J.R. Hayes, et al.; and the CLEERE Study Group. "Accommodative Lag before and after the Onset of Myopia." *Invest Ophthalmol Visual Sci* 47 (2006): E-Abstract 1166.

6. American Optometric Association (AOA). "Fourth Annual American Optometric Association American Eye-Q® Survey." The fourth annual American Eye-Q Survey was commissioned with Penn, Schoen & Berland Associates (PSB). From May 21–24, 2009, PSB interviewed 1,000 Americans, 18 years and older, representing a sample of the U.S. general population. (Margin of error for the survey: 95 percent confidence level.)

7. Sheedy, J.E. "Vision Problems at Video Display Terminals: A Survey of Optometrists." *J Am Optom Assoc* 63:10 (1992): 687–692.

8. American Optometric Association. "Recommended Eye Examination Frequency for Pediatric Patients and Adults." www.aoa.org/x5502.xml.

9. University of Illinois at Chicago, Department of Ophthalmology and Visual

Sciences. "Color Blindness." www.uic.edu/com/eye/LearningAboutVision/Eye-Facts/ColorBlindness.shtml.

10. Prevent Blindness America (formerly National Society to Prevent Blindness). *1993 Sports and Recreational Eye Injuries.* Schaumburg, IL: Prevent Blindness America, 1994.

11. Prevent Blindness America. "Sports Eye Safety." http://preventblindness.org/safety/sportspage1.html.

12. Prevent Blindness America. "Vision Problems in the U.S.-Prevalence of Adult Vision Impairment and Age-Related Eye Disease in America Report." Prevent Blindness America, 2002 edition. http://preventblindness.org.

13. Kaiser, H.J., J. Flammer, A. Schoetzau. "Blood Flow in Retrobulbar Vessels in Glaucoma Patients and Normals." In Drance, S.M. *Vascular Risk Factors and Neuroprotection in Glaucoma. Update 1996.* Amsterdam: Kugler, 1997, 135–138.

14. Gordon, M.O., J.A. Beiser, J.D. Brandt, et al.; for the Ocular Hypertension Treatment Study Group. "The Ocular Hypertension Treatment Study." *Arch Ophthalmol* 120 (2002): 714–720.

15. Thornton, J., R. Edwards, P. Mitchell, et al. "Smoking and Age-related Macular Degeneration: A Review of Association." *Eye* 19 (2005): 935–944.

16. VisionWatch data for six-month period ending December 2006. New York: Jobson Optical Research, 2007. www.jobsonresearch.com.

INDEX

About the Author

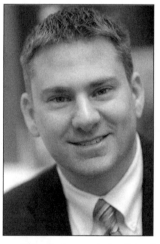

Dr. Joe Di Girolamo was born and raised in Southern California and his family later moved to Charlottesville, Virginia. He received his Bachelor's degree in biology from Villanova University. His graduate work at the Pennsylvania College of Optometry in Philadelphia included rotations through the Eye Institute in Philadelphia, the Omni Eye Center in Atlanta, and the Martinsburg Veteran's Administration Hospital. He graduated in 1996 and moved back to Virginia to join his father, also an optometrist, in practice. In 1998 he took over the practice, which today has multiple locations with several eye doctors on staff. Dr. Di Girolamo is a Remote Area Medical (RAM) volunteer optometrist and he also volunteers with the Optometry Giving Sight (OGS) nonprofit organization. He enjoys spending time with his family, reading, exercising, and GT auto racing. For more information, please visit his website: www.EyecareBook.com.